BISON
BOOKS

AT TABLE

A Taste of Heritage

Crow Indian Recipes & Herbal Medicines

ALMA HOGAN SNELL

Edited by
LISA CASTLE

Foreword by
KELLY KINDSCHER

UNIVERSITY OF NEBRASKA PRESS   LINCOLN & LONDON

All photographs are by Lisa M. Castle.

Library of Congress Cataloging-in-Publication Data
Snell, Alma Hogan.
A taste of heritage: Crow Indian recipes and herbal medicines /
Alma Hogan Snell; edited by Lisa Castle;
foreword by Kelly Kindsher.
p. cm.—(At table)
Includes bibliographical references and index.
ISBN-13: 978-0-8032-9353-3 (pbk.: alk. paper)
ISBN-10: 0-8032-9353-4 (pbk.: alk. paper)
1. Indian cookery. 2. Crow Indians—Food.
3. Medicinal plants. I. Castle, Lisa. II. Title.
III. At table series.
TX715.S669 2006
641.59'297—dc22   2006000821

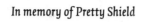

In memory of Pretty Shield

Contents

Illustrations

Foreword

Kelly Kindscher

In southern Montana, across the Crow Reservation, past fields of wheat and sugar beets, past cattle grazing on golden hills, past the St. Frances Xavier Mission and cabins rented to trout fisherman, and past the turnoff to the Yellowtail Dam, lies the Snell family home. I first drove there after my friend Robyn Klein told me that I needed to meet Alma Snell. Alma wanted to write a book on traditional Crow food recipes and herbal medicines, and she was looking for assistance. Much of my ethnobotanical work has involved studying and honoring Native American traditional knowledge, so I knew Robyn was right. I made arrangements to visit Alma at her home, nestled in the red sandstone foothills of the Big Horn Mountains and surrounded by ponderosa pines. I wanted to ask about her cookbook and tell her about Lisa Castle, a new graduate student who had come to work with me at the University of Kansas. Lisa had been an educator at the Denver Botanic Gardens, and I thought would likely be interested in helping with this project.

I hadn't been with Alma long before I realized that she is the most loving, positive person I have ever met. She was full of energy and determined to get her book published quickly because friends and relatives were already asking for it. I said that I would gladly help facilitate the book's coming together.

Alma supplied me with bison jerky and plum ketchup for the long trip back to Kansas. When I left, the evening light was golden on the mixed-grass prairie. I drove through the Crow Reservation and then south into the dark night of Wyoming. As I chewed on jerky topped with tasty plum sauce, I considered the work I would be doing in helping Alma publish her book.

Alma was taught the Crow traditions by her maternal grandmother, Pretty Shield. The knowledge gained from this education that was further influenced by her Christian upbringing, formal food-service training, and interest in herbalism makes Alma's understanding of foods and herbs unique and this book uniquely important.

Crow ethnobotany has not been widely shared and is not widely known. Although scattered references to the edible and medicinal uses of plants by the Crow exist, the first published work on uses of Crow plants was J. W. Blankinship's 1905 *Native Economic Plants of Montana*, which lists Crow uses for thirteen plants.[1] A more insightful work was written by a Crow woman, Joy Yellowtail Toineeta, whose 1970 master's thesis, titled *Absarog-Issawua (From the Land of the Crow Indians)*, is the most detailed ethnobotany of the Crow and discusses sixty-four species of plants.[2] Unfortunately, this work has never circulated beyond the few of us who have borrowed it from the Montana State University library. Jeff Hart, a Harvard graduate student, wrote *Montana—Native Plants and Early People* for a 1976 bicentennial book project.[3] He cataloged twenty-five Crow plants and their uses. Together these three works form the heart of the previously published record of Crow ethnobotany.

Outside of publications, it is well known that the Crows have a rich tradition of plant use. Because generations of the Crow people have inhabited their lands continuously, this information is steeped in cultural heritage. Alma reveals many unique uses of plants from the Crow tradition that have never been written about. More important than listing the kinds of plants used by the Crows, she provides detailed recipes showing how these plants were and are used to make foods and medicines (with modern updates). Alma Snell's book offers us an important glimpse into the history and significance of Crow ethnobotany.

Notes

1. J. W. Blankinship, *Native Economic Plants of Montana* (Montana Agricultural College Experiment Station, Bulletin 56, 1905): 3–36.

2. Joy Yellowtail Toineeta, "Absarog-Issawua (From the Land of the Crow Indians)" (master's thesis, Montana State University, 1970).

3. Jeff Hart, *Montana—Native Plants and Early Peoples* (Helena: The Montana Historical Society, 1976).

Acknowledgments

The knowledge contained in this book has been gleaned from count-less elders who have shared and helped me wherever I have been. Not only have I learned from Grandma Pretty Shield and other Crow el-ders but also from Lena Blue Robe Snell, One Woman Buck, and other Assiniboine elders and people from all across the Great Plains. This learning continues as my sisters and Eloise Pease, Annie Walks, and so many others keep surprising me with new information. Thanks to you all.

The making of this book has led to many pleasant reminiscences about the old days from people all over the community. To the many of you who have shared stories with me, I am grateful not only for the knowledge but also for the chance to share laughter and friend-ship. *A ho.*

This book crosses disciplinary boundaries between traditional knowledge, herbalism, cooking, and botany and brings aspects of them together. Many experts in each of these fields have given their expertise (and sometimes their books) to me. Thanks go to Robyn Klein (the first modern herbalist I've really known), Kelly Kindscher, Bonnie Heidl, Bob Krumm, Thomas Elpel, and so many others.

Nature provides many plants, but without my family, the Grangers, Fort Belknap cousins of my husband Bill, and other helpful harvest-ers, the turnips would still be in the ground and the berries on the bushes. Thanks for picking the plants and bringing them to me.

The interest of my family members and their willingness to help me pick berries, dig roots, and prepare for programs have helped immensely. They have also been willing to eat my wild foods and take my wild remedies, even when they haven't been sure what's in them. Without the lifelong support of my husband, Bill Snell, none of this would have been possible.

I'd also like to thank all the audiences at my presentations and the readers of this book. Your enthusiasm and ideas have helped me continue my work, knowing that people are interested in walking with nature and learning what she has to say.

I (Lisa, the editor) wish to thank Hillary Loring, Maggie Riggs, and Peggy Castle for painstaking readings of manuscript drafts; Robyn Klein for the roundabout introduction to Alma Snell; the friends, family, and coworkers at the Kansas Biological Survey who have enthusiastically supported my annual cross-country jaunts; and my parents, who have encouraged me in everything but especially my passionate pursuit of plant knowledge—ever since I started eating snails in their garden at age two. Kelly Kindscher has been the background support behind the project, providing introductions, information, plant identifications, advice, and friendship. Most especially, thanks to Alma and Bill Snell for opening their house and hearts to me.

Finally, from all of us involved with this project, all thanks to the Creator.

Editor's Introduction

Few cookbooks have characters. Even fewer plant books do. But this book distinctly does. It is not an ordinary cookbook nor an ordinary plant book. It is an extraordinary combination of wild plant knowledge, historical and modern recipes, natural medicine, and advice for life. It is written by an extraordinary woman, and the people who influenced her can hardly be considered ordinary either. Together they compose the characters of this book.

Throughout the book, we read of Alma Snell's grandmother, Pretty Shield. A Crow medicine woman who lived from 1856 to 1944 and survived the tumultuous changes in Crow Indian society, Pretty Shield raised Alma (and many of her other grandchildren) after Alma's mother, Helen Goes Ahead, died in 1924 when Alma was only one year old.

In this book, we see Pretty Shield as she is often portrayed. She is the proud widow of Goes Ahead, who was a distinguished Crow warrior who scouted for the U.S. Army at the time of General Custer. She is also the powerful midwife who eased pain with her plants and the great storyteller who shared her life story with anthropologist Frank Linderman. We also view the personal side of Pretty Shield. We see a woman who acknowledges the power of the ants around her, a woman who carries her digger out to the field to unearth the turnips at their freshest, a woman who boils her coffee strong. We realize that for all the knowledge that Pretty Shield passed on to Alma, for which we are grateful, the greatest thing that Pretty Shield gave her is love. That love is returned, and it infuses Alma's stories.

Alma's husband, Bill Snell, is critical to the story in this book. Whether as a rancher, marine, or law enforcement officer, Bill has put in full days of hard work all his life, and he expects the same of others. Within a few moments spent with this soft-spoken man, one senses a great depth of kindness, intelligence, and devotion. Alma explains that she never would have continued giving her Taste of Heritage programs, upon which this book is based, without the constant support of Bill. These days he carries her boxes of "weeds" and smiles at the constant stream of visitors who find their house in the foothills of the Big Horn Mountains in southern Montana. He tests her new wild-food recipes with good humor but still prefers a simple piece of huckleberry pie.

Watching Alma and Bill together, one can clearly see why lonesome or troubled people come to Alma, the "Love Mama," for relationship advice. Throughout their fifty-plus years of marriage, she and Bill seem to have figured out a great partnership. Alma says that Bill's love of planting and gardening along with her love of wild plants contributes to their togetherness.

Often Alma's four children and twelve grandchildren show up in these stories. One of them is always having some sort of an adventure. Alma always seems to know how to help out, whether with cookies and conversation, prayers and advice, or tincture and bandages.

Alma has established herself in many circles that extend far beyond the confines of southern Montana. First it was Bill's career that took the couple across the country. Then it became Alma's presentations. Now this spry eighty-year-old seems to know everybody. She's helped people with the National Park Service, the Smithsonian Institution, the Frontier House project of the Public Broadcasting Service, the Montana Herb Gathering, and the Billy Graham Crusade, to name just a few, so it shouldn't be a surprise that she is well connected. Alma has continued to both share and learn wherever she goes. She learns botanical information from those she describes as "the best in the business." She continues to excitedly glean information from "experts," like herbalist Robyn Klein, ethnobotanist Kelly Kindscher, and berry man Bob Krumm, while sharing with them joy, knowledge, and sometimes medicine.

Alma mentions me on a few pages. A graduate student working on a doctorate in biology, I feel blessed to have been involved in this project. Plants, food, people, and words all enthrall me, so our collaboration has been a serendipitously good fit. Through a stroke of good fortune, my study organism, the wild turnips Alma so loves to dig, grow right across the road from the Snell household. I was able to spend part of the last four summers working with Alma, watching her presentations and traipsing over the red hills with Bill's beloved golden retriever, Penny.

Despite all these incidental characters, one person is really at the center of this work: Alma Hogan Snell herself. Alma possesses a unique combination of traditional knowledge and formal education along with healing gifts and culinary skills. Her willingness to share these gifts makes her an author like no other. While many of the recipes and plant uses are representative of Native American life on the Great Plains, Alma's stories are all personal. She did not just hear an elder tell her to use a plant in a certain way; she has found that plant, dug it up, and administered it as needed. Alma loves the foods of her ancestors, but when she thinks that bay leaves make a better stew seasoning than mint leaves (even though bay is exotic and mint grows wild in Crow country), she'll adjust the recipe. Alma knows that Crow culture is active, vibrant, and ever changing. Her recipes and stories reflect this.

As of this writing, Alma is an astoundingly active eighty-two years old. She constantly fields phone calls from those in need of healing, makes tea for whomever stops by, and shares her love and knowledge through words. She moves from Crow to English with ease and silently sends messages across the room using Indian Sign Language. The kind of woman who says her prayers as the sun rises (well before 5 a.m. in Montana in summer), Alma is a woman with long-term goals. Whenever I visit she has a new plan for what is going to happen next. She might start writing children's novels. She might change the topic of her public presentations. She might just finish all the needlework and beadwork projects she has started over the years. She has the skill and desire for all these projects. She just needs to find the time. Whatever she does, Alma will not be sitting still for long.

Reading these recipes and plant uses, Alma's gifts are evident. Not only endowed with cooking and healing skills, she is an accomplished storyteller with a sense of humor. Enjoy.

Author's Introduction

My grandmother Pretty Shield, a good, loving, powerful, full-blooded Crow Indian woman, raised me. With great courage and love she taught me the ways of our people. She taught me to cook, nurture, heal, and so much more. To this day when I am in a reminiscing spirit, I hear Grandma's voice, strong as ever, caring as always, "Don't forget what I have taught you. Words are powerful. Keep them in your heart and tell them to others who you feel will benefit from them."

Readers, I hope that you will benefit from Pretty Shield's words and from mine as well. In this book, I have collected wild plant information, recipes, stories of healing, and advice about love, beauty, and life. Much of the information comes straight from Pretty Shield. Other bits I have learned through my eighty-odd years on this earth. I pray it will be of use to you.

My ancestors, especially the gifted ones, could tell what is wrong with a person by talking to and observing him or her. Many, like Grandma, had an uncanny sense for what to do. Such a sense was a gift. By the time I was born in Crow Agency, Montana, in 1923, Grandma had become a Christian and settled into reservation life. Still, she had a great memory of the time when the Crow followed the buffalo and powerful knowledge of healing and the world around her.[1] When friends of my generation were off learning "modern" cooking and sewing at classes on the reservation, Pretty Shield was taking me out to collect plants.

I have also been blessed with many other knowledgeable elders in my life. When I married Bill Snell in 1947, I spent time with his Assiniboine family further north in Montana.[2] I learned from them many new uses of plants, many recipes, and many common household tasks. As my husband's career advanced, we had the opportunity to live on reservations throughout the West. Wherever we went, I started seeking out the old women and learning from them. Even when I was a very young woman, I wanted to know what the elders had to say. Pretty Shield had taught me so much, and I knew that other old people could too. Many of their stories, recipes, and cures have become my own, and I have included them in this book.

So my recipes and my knowledge come from many sources. I have had jobs—from working in food service in a hospital to serving at a fancy restaurant to running my own café—that have taught me more about food. I've learned from formal training. I've learned from books and articles and the many experts who hear about me and come to talk to me way back here on the Crow Reservation in Montana. Many times I have learned just from trying something. But no matter how they come to me, I know that my knowledge and healing power come from the Lord.

When I am called to help with healing, I feel the guidance of the Spirit of God to know what to do. By obedience and faith I have been proof of the power of the creation of God in its natural ways. All the same, I thank God for medical science to do marvelous things to the human body. God bless the doctors, nurses, researchers, and caregivers. We are all working together.

In much the same way, I am glad for supermarkets and many modern conveniences. While nature provides for those who know where to look, strict adherence to the "old ways" just because they are old seems foolish to me. When Grandma had a chance to replace her wooden digging stick with one made of wrought iron, she did. She went with what worked better. I am not going to spend all day pounding roots with rocks when I have a food processor that works wonders.

Yet in this modern world we still have a lot to learn from tradition. I feel there is value in our Crow foods and medical substances that can ward off many sicknesses. If we practice our ancestors' way of preparing food and living healthfully, we may be able to prevent a lot of ills.

Notes

1. Many of Pretty Shield's stories can be found in a book by Frank Linderman, *Pretty-Shield: Medicine Woman of the Crows*.

2. I wrote details about my life with Pretty Shield, my turbulent courtship with Bill, and the early years of our marriage in my autobiography *Grandmother's Grandchild: My Crow Indian Life*, which was edited by Becky Matthews and published by the University of Nebraska Press in 2000.

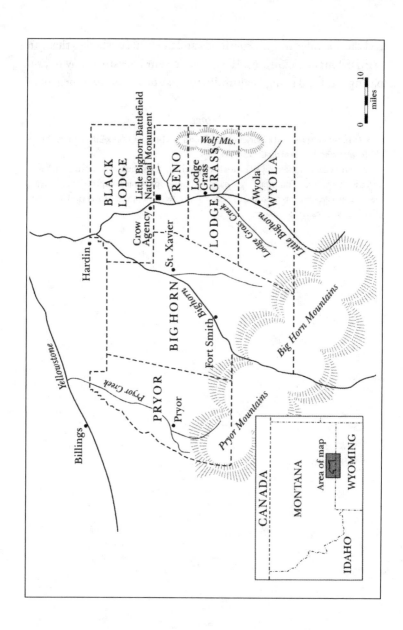

Crow Reservation

A TASTE OF HERITAGE

PART ONE

A Taste of Heritage Foods

A Vision of Cooking

Food is something I seem destined to care about. In fact, my gift with food came to me after my grandmother Pretty Shield had a vision about it when I was very young.

In her dream there was a young woman in the middle of a stream. Then an older woman appeared on the side of the stream, and she told Pretty Shield that these were gifts: beading and cooking. She should give them to her granddaughters. Pretty Shield had already decided to give the gifts to Cerise, my oldest sister, and me. Since she was the oldest, Cerise got to choose first. She chose beading, so I got cooking.

All my life I've ended up around the food, cooking. I didn't always start there. In the hospital I started as an aide, but then I was helping out in the kitchen, and they saw what I could do there, so they had me stay. Later I worked in restaurants. Then, at Pine Ridge, I was the supervisor of food service. No matter where I've been, I've been around food. That's my gift.

Cerise is a great beader. The best. If you ever see a piece of beadwork done by Cerise Stewart, pay whatever they're asking. It's worth it. She truly has a gift.

But, I've always been kind of glad that she chose beading. That left the food for me.

Even though I have had years of experience in food service (in fact I completed the Indian Health Food Service Supervisor course at the head of my class), I have written this book from a lodgekeeper's standpoint. The lodgekeeper, or homemaker, has always been a very important role in Crow society. The size of my family is always changing. Sometimes it is just my husband and me; sometimes one of my twelve grandchildren will come by; sometimes it is the whole tribe at a celebration or feed; and sometimes I feel that the whole of humanity is my family as I try to teach the world through my programs. However big my family is, I am happy to cook for them. Providing family members with food is more than just giving them nutrients—it is creating a home for them, keeping the lodge.

So these recipes are not formally tested in spotless lab kitchens in big cities. They are recipes that I have served as a lodgekeeper for my family. You'll want to try them out with yours.

Plant Foods

Walking with Nature

When you look around Crow Country, it can be hard to believe that there was ever enough to eat out there. Lots of times there wasn't much, but nature did provide. My grandmother taught me how the Crow people walked with nature throughout the year. They walked with nature and nature provided. People ate everything in its time, and I think they were healthier for it.

At the end of winter, when everyone was running out of dried meat, berries, and roots, springtime would come around and provide what you needed, just as you needed it.

Bread food and brain food come first. In June, here is this wild turnip. We call it *ehe*. It is our bread, and it will fill you up after a long winter. Also the bitterroot comes in June. That's a mind health food.

Soon the berries come in, one after the other. They provide vitamin C. Of course we didn't know they had vitamin B, vitamin C, or whatever, but they were there, and the berries were ready, and we ate them. Nature was actually saying, "Come, you need this. So eat this now and preserve the rest of it for this winter." And we go along, and here come the grapes. Oh, they're ready! Nature says, "Eat."

And so we eat. What we can't eat right then, we put away for winter. Then we go to another phase, to plums, for example. Plums come along and say, "You have had your roots and berries. Now your body needs plums. Here are plums." If nature could only speak right out to us, she'd say, "This is what this contains, and you need it in your body." Nature can't talk directly to us, so she ripens what we need just in time for us to eat it.

I do believe that nature provides at each step along the way. We never had all this year-round choice of food as we do now. We had each thing in its season. We walked with nature. Nature provided, and we were healthy.

The stories and recipes in this section should help you use wild food plants and take your own walk with nature.

Wild Vegetables

The plant foods in this section are arranged by season, in the order that nature provides them each year, and by importance.

Wild Turnip: Ehe

Pediomelum esculentum
Prairie Turnip, Breadroot, Scurf Pea, Timpsula

Ehe, wild turnips—they are our bread food. Of course our turnips are different from garden turnips. Ehe doesn't taste or look like garden turnips, and botanists tell me that it is not even related to them. The plant I am talking about is a little perennial that grows out on the prairie (some call it prairie turnip) with leaves that look like little hands with five fingers. The little purple flowers you notice only if you are looking at just the right time. It's a fuzzy plant, furry on both the stems and blossoms. The scientists used to call it *Psoralea esculenta*, but now they tell me the Latin name is *Pediomelum esculentum*.

Ehe roots are covered with a thick brown bark. The part of the root that you eat is about the size of a chicken egg, sometimes smaller. It has a flat yet distinctive taste that is all its own. It is sweet when it first comes out of the ground, especially the young ones. Later it tastes a little like field corn, if you've ever chewed on a kernel of field corn. Some say wild turnips taste like raw green beans or unroasted peanuts. Others think they are just bland. Turnips make a nice gruel for babies and sick people, and they are good for bread, of course, and thickening. They dry very well, which is why they were so important to the Crow people. You can dry the roots and braid them together and always have some sustenance to get you through the winter.

Finding and Digging Wild Turnips

Wild turnips are usually ready in June. It's a chore to spot them, dig them up, and store them, but we as a family think they are worth it. Back when I was growing up, living with my grandmother, we'd spend a few days doing nothing but digging turnips. My sister Pearl, Grandma, and I would bring home three hundred or more roots. We stayed in the turnip area all day. We took our lunch. It was hard work, but we liked it.

More recently (I think it was two years ago), I went out doing some serious digging. My son Bill Junior and his wife, Karen, went with me, and we dug about 250 roots. That sounds like a lot, but that's not very many if you want to make a wreath or carry a family through the winter. Fortunately, we have always been able to buy potatoes and flour, so we were never dependent on just the turnips. Pretty Shield always seemed to collect just enough, so she would usually have a few left when spring came along.

To find wild turnips, look on rocky slopes that aren't overly grazed. I always look for a slope that comes gently down to the level. There have to be a few rocks where they like to grow. When I was young I used to wish that you'd find turnips in a smooth, gardenlike place with soft soil. But it doesn't happen. I believe that those roots grow down pretty far in the gravel. They can reach any moisture they need and the rocks seem to help trap it in there. So look on rocky slopes.

Turnips wedge themselves in the ground, and you have to dig quite deep to get them out. Turnip digging sticks were traditionally made from chokecherry wood. They were made in the same way as arrows, except without the arrowhead. Chokecherry is sturdy, straight, and semihard. A man would shave off the bark, hold the stick over hot coals, and keep rolling and shaping it until it was baked through and straight. You had to do all the twisting and straightening before the heating because the sticks were hard as rock when they were done. Later the government came with its blacksmiths, and they made iron diggers. They were faster and easier to use. That's what Pretty Shield used while I was growing up. Now my son uses a long spade when we go out digging.

Whatever tool you use, digging turnips is hard work. The fat part of the root isn't that close to the surface, and you want to get a nice long tail of the taproot with it. You have to get all around the plant with your digger and loosen the earth so that you can stick your shovel in there and work it up. That way you can pull out the root easily, and the earth remains in the hole. You have to put the earth back. Put the earth back that you have taken out with your shovel, so animals won't step in the hole. Then you cut off the top of the plant and leave it to tumble in the wind, for the seed to spread.

Wild Turnip Confusion with Lupine

Be careful when you dig turnips that you don't confuse them with lupine (*Lupinus* species), which they resemble. Lupine is poisonous. When you dig turnips all your life, you know exactly what they look like. One could be sitting right in the middle of a patch of lupine, and those who don't know the wild turnip probably won't see it, but experienced turnip diggers would eye it immediately. We'd know what it was.

I remember a young man over at Fort Belknap who gathered some turnips for his aunt. He went out and gathered a bunch of them for his aunt, who is my friend and can't see very well. He brought the turnips to her, and she was looking and feeling around and looking real close, as much as she could with her poor eyes. And she said, "This is not turnip." Some roots, she said, almost smelled something like turnips, but she knew they weren't right. "I knew it wasn't turnip, so I didn't eat it. I didn't fix it. So I threw them out." Later on we found out that they were lupine. So somebody didn't know too much about turnips.

A TASTE OF HERITAGE FOODS

Cleaning and Storing Wild Turnips

As soon as you dig some turnips, bring them home. They must be peeled quickly, as the tough outer skin is leathery and must be ripped off the vegetable as soon as possible. If they're not peeled right away, the turnips will need to be soaked and messed with, and that is definitely not a pleasant undertaking.

Shake off any clods of dirt you have left on your turnips and take a good look. The roots have little branching growths on them. If you can grasp one of those and pull back on it, then your fingernails have a chance of getting in there and pulling the bark off. Otherwise you start at the long tail of the root, and you peel the bark away toward the fat part, which is what you will eat. That's the way Grandma told us how to do it. It's easier to pull down to the head of the turnip than it is to pull the other way, from head to tail.

If you have a great deal of turnips, you can braid those big long root tails together. If you have a very great deal of them, you can just keep adding turnips to the braid until it is big enough to make a wreath or a door decoration. Then put a ribbon on it and hang it up.

Pretty Shield never did that. For storing them, she either slivered the roots and dried them on a tarp or hung them up whole to dry. If you hang them up whole to dry, then you also put them in the pot whole. After you boil dried turnips for a while, they become soft enough that you can get a hold of them, cut them in half, and take the middle core out. Turnips have a stringy core that is usually kind of hard to eat and chew. When I was growing up, Pretty Shield would put the dried turnips in a cloth sack so there would be air flow but they would be kept dry and clean at the same time.

For chipping turnips, Pretty Shield used a large canvas tarp. She'd lay the canvas down on the ground, and she'd place her rock in the middle of it. She'd sit on one side of the rock with her mallet, and she'd pound away at the turnips. If the pieces scattered, they would stay on the cloth. She always collected the scraps in the tarp after she had finished her work. She scraped them toward the rock, and then she put them in her root bag. Today I chop the roots in my food processor and store them in airtight containers. Whole dried turnip roots I store in cloth bags.

After a summer of hard digging and drying, we had in our storeroom the chipped kind, the mashed-up kind, and whole roots. If you leave them whole, the taste seems to be preserved much better. But it's so much easier to grab a handful of slivered ones and throw them into a stew. Both ways you can make a good stew, but if you really like the taste, then leave them whole.

The Best Wild Turnips

Even though the biggest turnips are the most fun to find, they are not the best tasting. The young, thin ones have the best taste. They are sweet and crisp and really good to eat fresh. Later on, when they're old and husky, they start to get knots and wrinkles on the outside, and the insides taste like wood. You eat them because you kind of adjust yourself to that taste. These old turnips can still be used in soups, but they're not very good used as is, as a vegetable, because they are spongy. They're like chewing on soft wood or even rubber. There is no moisture in them. You can't bite through one unless you pound it with something sharp and separate it from its core and cook it and cook it until tender.

We have had to eat some of those old hard roots when the turnips were not so plentiful. We'd use the hard ones first and save the good ones, the thin ones, for later.

Too Many Wild Turnips

Eating too many turnips can create a lot of gas in the digestive system. Then you have to drink mint tea to take it down. They can also cause constipation, which Pretty Shield always warned us against. "Don't eat too much, or you're going to get clogged up, and we'll have problems."

❧ Wild Turnip Flour and Turnip Meal

Several recipes call for turnip flour or turnip meal. In either case, all you need are dried turnips, some rocks, and a lot of patience—or a good food processor.

Take dried turnips and grind them to a fine powder for flour. Make the powder a little coarser, like the consistency of cornmeal, if you are going to use it for porridge.

❧ Wild Turnip Porridge

This warming porridge is easy on the stomach, so it is frequently fed to convalescing people and babies. It also makes a hearty breakfast.

2 cups ground turnip meal
2 to 3 cups warm water
Flour
2 tablespoons marrow fat or other shortening
Sugar to taste

Soak the ground turnip meal in warm water in a saucepan until the particles are soft and swollen. Let simmer over medium heat until the meal is tender, about half an hour. Mix the flour with enough water to make a smooth paste (about 3 scant tablespoons of flour to 1 cup of water). Add to the cooked turnip. Stir vigorously to prevent lumping. Cover and boil for 5 minutes. Add marrow fat or shortening and remove from the fire. This is best sweetened with a little sugar and served warm.

Serves about six adults. Use good judgment in serving this porridge to convalescing people and babies.

❧ Wild Turnip Bread

    3 cups all-purpose flour
    1 cup turnip flour
    2 tablespoons or 2 packages yeast
    2 teaspoons salt
    4 tablespoons soft shortening
    2 1/2 cups warm water
    2 to 4 tablespoons sugar (optional)

    Combine all-purpose flour, turnip flour, yeast, and salt and mix well
    with an electric mixer or hand whip. Add the shortening and warm wa-
    ter. Add 2 to 4 tablespoons of sugar, if desired. Mix well with the mixer
    or turn out on a floured board and knead for at least twenty minutes.
    Let rise for one hour. Then punch down, work the dough well between
    your hands, and form into loaves. Place the dough in greased loaf pans
    and let rise again for about an hour. Bake at 350 degrees for one hour.

    Makes 3 medium or 2 large loaves of bread.

The only time I ever did think of visiting another country was
when I was digging turnips. I thought I must be getting pretty close
to China.

Bitterroot: Basauxawa

Lewisia rediviva

Basauxawa, bitterroot, is nature's great mind food that comes in the
spring. This little plant grows high in the mountains and has beautiful pink flowers. But you don't use the top part—it's horribly bitter.
You eat the little roots. The Crow name means "lots of veins" or "bushy
limbs"; that describes the roots as they go here and there and everywhere. The English name describes the taste.

Bitterroot is for clearing up the mind. Crow people (and other
Plains Indians) are an oral people. All our knowledge was kept in the
mind and passed down from generation to generation through stories and songs. We depend on our memory. Bitterroot gives clarity
and improves memory. Men especially like to eat it because they want

A TASTE OF HERITAGE FOODS

to tell stories and remember better, and they need their heads to be clear to do that.

Women like to take bitterroot because they have so much to do, especially when they are beading and watching children and really need to concentrate. It works very well. Everything looks brighter. You can breathe better. It feels as if you have a clear head. I take a few bites when I'm going to give a demonstration. It doesn't take much.

You can chew on dried roots (they're easy to break off with your teeth) but most often bitterroot is cooked. Usually we sauce it: cook it and mix in a little cornstarch for thickening and a little sugar for sweetness.

After the roots are dried you can use them all year long, but mostly we eat bitterroot when nature provides it in June. We seem to always have a kind of craving for it then, for that taste. You suddenly go about looking for someone who has it: "Oh, I'm hungry for bitterroot." Sometimes you need this special mind food.

Harvest and Preparation

Bitterroot is harvested in the bud by using a small hand shovel or knife. Just as soon as the roots are dug up, they should be placed in a pan of water, so the bark can be gently slipped off. Placing the clean roots on a tarp in a dry place out of the direct sun is the best way to dry them.

In the old days, if we came to a big patch of a plant like bitterroot, we'd always leave behind about one third of them. We never counted, but it usually worked out to be about a third of the plants. Then, if somebody else came to that patch, and they would see that most of it was gone, they wouldn't touch what's there, and they would go and dig somewhere else. Back then bitterroot was easy to find, but now you have to travel to get any.

Botanists tell me that bitterroot is becoming scarce, so I don't recommend that you dig it now.

🍂 Brain Healthy Porridge: Wild Bitterroot Sauce

This sauce is usually served on its own rather than poured over something, and it makes enough for 6 to 8 people—a small saucerful for each person.

2 cups cleaned whole bitterroots
6 cups water
5 tablespoons cornstarch
²/₃ cup sugar
Dried wild grapes or raisins (optional)

Place the bitterroots in the water in a saucepan and boil for 45 minutes, or until tender. Add the cornstarch and sugar to thicken. Continue cooking, stirring constantly, until thick. Serve warm. Dried wild grapes or raisins can be sprinkled on just before serving, if desired.

Wild Onions: Bitxua

Allium textile and other Allium species

The prairie onion, that's my specialty. It has a skin that looks like burlap, but remove the skin and that prairie onion is white and clean and nutritious. Prairie onions have a garlic taste to them, and just as it does with garlic, the smell lingers with you.

My grandma Pretty Shield always said, "Eat some of these; these are good for you." She'd throw a handful or half a handful into stew. She liked the onions cooked, but I remember now and then seeing her nibble on a raw one, straight from the ground.

There is another edible wild onion around here, the nodding onion (Allium cernuum). I have never paid too much attention to it, but the Flatheads use the nodding onion a lot. These onions taste just fine, but they don't have the strong garlic flavor of our wild prairie onion.

Wild Carrot: Bikka:sahte

Perideridia gairdneri
Split Root, Yampa, Squaw Root

Wild carrot: split root, we call it. Others call it yampa or squaw root. The botanists call it Perideridia gairdneri. Whatever you call it, wild carrot roots are a taste treat.

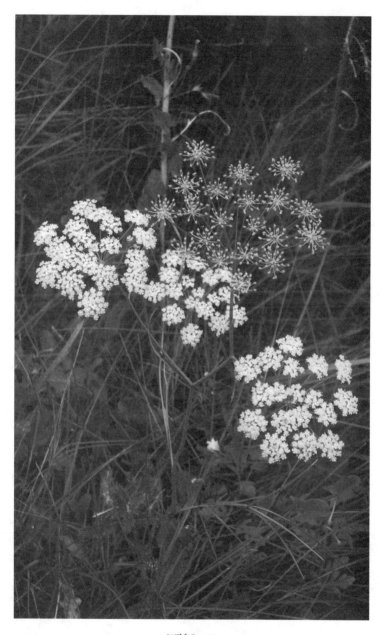

Wild Carrot

This delicate little plant with ferny leaves and white flowers grows up high in the mountains. You won't find any down in the valley, and in the foothills you'll find them only in damp places, if you are lucky. Up high in the mountains they grow in open meadows, sometimes acres and acres of them, but usually they're just here and there.

I like to eat them as is, raw. I don't care too much about them cooked. They are fine boiled with a little sugar, but I prefer them raw in salads. I like split root in salads because it's crunchy and nice. They're good in stews too. I like to add them to dried-meat or rabbit stew. I just throw in a bunch of the roots because they taste so much like carrots. Wild carrots really season the stew.

Harvesting Wild Carrots

Around here wild carrots can be ready in June. The last part of June is probably the best time, but you can dig them well into July. We dig the mature plants as we see them. While we're harvesting, younger plants will just be starting, so we dig wild carrots many times from the first harvest to the last. If the season lasts quite a while, we dig them until they are through. Right at the point where the stem connects to the root the plants are very, very delicate. They can break off easily, so you must be careful digging them. The stem can break off and fall, and then you won't know where your carrot is. You need to get the root and the plant while they are connected. It takes some practice to dig them right.

When I was young, we often dug wild carrots in the Wolf Mountains, and when we came over here to the Big Horns, to pick berries or something, we'd dig them then. It was during our berry-picking trips that we'd find them. Now I just have to drive uphill from my house, and I'll see bunches of them scattered around.

You can dry wild carrots, but they'll always shrivel to a much smaller size when they are completely dry. To dry carrots, scatter them on a tarp and sun dry them. They will dry in three or four days.

Wild carrots are not as plentiful as they were some fifty years ago. If you can't find them or don't want to dig them because there aren't many near you, you can substitute domestic carrots in all of the recipes that call for them.

Editor's Note: Split root (*Perideridia gairdneri*) is not the same plant as Queen Anne's Lace (*Daucus carota*), which is also called wild carrot. While the roots look and taste somewhat different, both can be used in these recipes. Be aware, however, that the carrot family also contains many poisonous plants, including poison hemlock. Know your plants well before eating them.

❧ Wild Carrot Pudding

   2 cups whole wild carrots
   2 cups water, approximately
   2 tablespoons sugar
   2 tablespoons flour (wild turnip flour or regular all-purpose wheat flour)

   Cover the carrots with water and cook in a saucepan until tender. Add the sugar. Add the flour by first making it into a paste with a little water and then stirring it into the simmering carrots until thick. Remove from the heat and eat warm.
   Serves 4 as a side dish.

Cattails: Baxosa
Typha species

"If you live near a marsh, you need never go hungry," I tell lots of school groups, and it's true.

If you live anywhere near a wet place, you probably live near a great food plant. Cattails grow in wetlands and marshes all over the country. Surprisingly, they are a great source of protein, and all parts, from the tender shoots to the insides of the roots to the young fruits and even the flowers and pollen are edible.

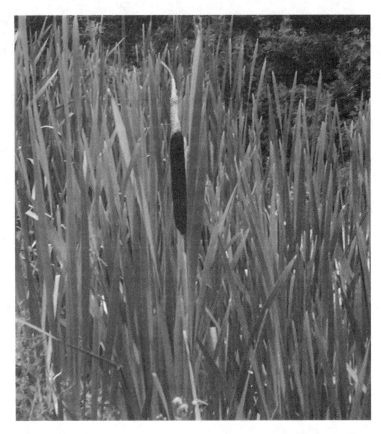

Cattails

❧ Fresh Wild Salad

As a boy my husband, Bill, and his friends would pull out shoots of cattail stalks and eat them just as is. Bill says they seemed sweet to him. The tender stalks these days can be diced and mixed with other salad vegetables.

> 1 cup tender cattail stalks, diced
> 2 handfuls watercress, well washed
> 8 wild carrot roots, cleaned (leave whole or dice the large roots)
> 1 handful yucca blossoms
> 1 tablespoon cattail seeds (gathered from the very tip of the spike before it turns to fluff)

A TASTE OF HERITAGE FOODS

Toss together the cattail stalk pieces, watercress, wild carrots, and yucca blossoms. Sprinkle the cattail seeds over all. Serve with your favorite dressing. (My favorite dressing for this salad is made with equal amounts of wild grape juice and cherry wine vinegar and enough olive oil to sprinkle over the whole salad.)

Serves 4.

Cattail Biscuits

Assiniboine women used to wade out in the shallow water of a marsh in their bare feet. That way they could find with their toes the thick, fattened parts of the cattail rhizomes. They'd reach down and dig out that fat bulblike piece. I've made flour from the center of the root that grows straight down too. Either way, to make flour take the roots or rhizomes, dry them, and then grind them up for flour. The old way to make flour was to grind the roots between rocks over a tarp to catch the pieces, but I always use my food processor. Cattail roots and rhizomes are very nutritious and for a plant food high in protein.

These biscuits taste somewhat like they're made with rye flour.

2 cups cattail root flour
1 tablespoon cattail seeds
2 cups whole-wheat flour
4 teaspoons baking powder
1 1/4 cups milk
2/3 cup canola oil

Mix all the ingredients together well. Use your hands to shape the dough into disks about 3 inches in diameter and just under an inch thick. Place on a cookie sheet and bake at 450 degrees for about 10 minutes, or until golden brown. Serve with your favorite jam.

Yields about 8 or 10 biscuits.

ࣿ Buffalo Cattail Stew

> 1 pound fresh buffalo meat (or other meat), cut into pieces
> 6 cups water
> 1 bay leaf (optional)
> 1 cup cattail stalks or roots, chopped
> 1 cup cornmeal
> 5 cedar berries (optional; sold in stores as "juniper berries," from
>   the *Juniperus* species)
> Salt and pepper

Place the meat in a 2-quart saucepan. Add water to two inches above the top of the meat. Toss in the bay leaf (if you prefer the taste of bay leaf). Cook over medium heat for 2 hours. Add the cattail, cornmeal, and cedar berries (if you like the flavor of cedar berries; otherwise skip these and use the bay leaf instead—choose one or the other but don't use both). Continue to cook, stirring regularly, until the cornmeal is cooked. Add salt and pepper to taste.

Yucca: Oox'ish bautshua

Yucca glauca

Even though they look intimidating (the Crow name means "deer's awl," and they are sharp), yucca plants are surprisingly useful. Fresh yucca flowers, especially the petals, are a treat to eat. The flavor is a little sweet and a little nutty and very clean. Yucca flowers and pods can be cooked a little too, but I think they are best fresh in salads or other dishes. Cows and ants also really like to eat yucca, so make sure the flowers are fresh and ant free before you pick them.

Salsify: Ba boba sheeb dauxa

Tragopogon dubius
Oyster Plant, Goatsbeard

Salsify is a weed that grows on the hills around here. The seedhead looks like a giant dandelion puff after it blooms. Just before the seeds all blow away, I like to pick the seedheads and spray them with hairspray. They make nice additions to dried flower arrangements, and

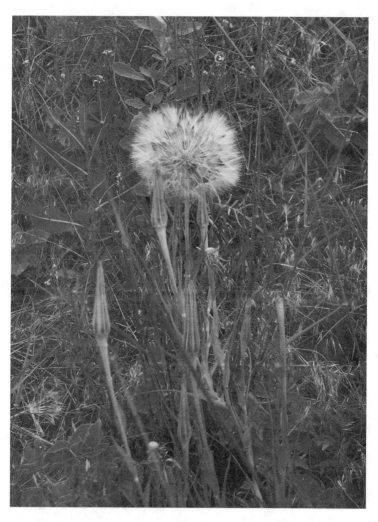

Salisfy

these days I pick them for their seedheads more often than I dig them for food. Still, the roots can be eaten, and some say they taste like oysters. Here's a poor man's salsify stew recipe if you want to try for yourself.

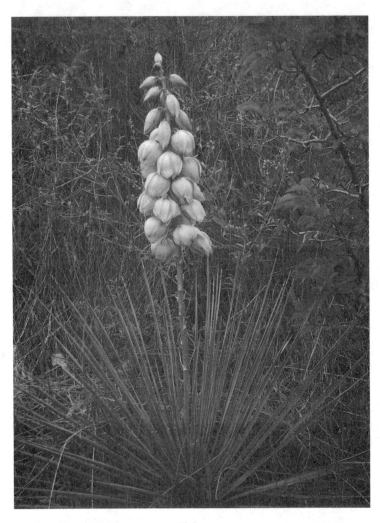

Yucca

A TASTE OF HERITAGE FOODS

⚖ Salsify Oyster Stew

12 salsify roots
2 potatoes, diced
6 cups water (or just enough to cover substance)
1 teaspoon salt
¹/₄ teaspoon black pepper or shepherd's purse seeds
3 cups milk
1 cup cream
2 tablespoons butter

Dig the oyster plants in the summer when the plants are in full bloom. Take the roots of about a dozen plants, wash them, scrape them, and chop them into pieces 1 inch long. Place the chopped roots and diced potatoes into hot water that has been seasoned with salt and black pepper or shepherd's purse. Cook until the roots are tender. Combine the milk and cream and heat separately but do not scald. Place the roots, potatoes, and cooking liquid in a blender on the chop cycle for 1 minute. Turn the root mixture into a serving dish, add butter and the hot milk mixture, and serve.

Serves 4.

Ground Tomato: Bitgup awada
Physalis pumila
Wild Tomatillo, Husk Tomato, Ground Cherry

The ground tomato is a little weed you see creeping up alongside roads or in fields. After taking off the tan-colored husk, you'll see the orange-red berry inside. It was usually eaten just as is, but some mixed it with foods that needed a little sweetening. I have never tried baking with it, but a tourist once spied some ground tomatoes growing on our property and told me that she had baked a pie with them and that it was very good. I didn't get her recipe, but I imagine the fruit boiled, thickened, and flavored with cinnamon, ginger, or orange juice.

ᔧ Ground Tomato Salad

This modern recipe makes a cooling summer side dish.

> 1 pound of husked ground tomatoes
> 1 tablespoon olive oil
> 1 tablespoon vinegar
> 1 cucumber, sliced
> Salt and pepper

Mix together all the ingredients. Chill until ready to serve.

Wild Asparagus: Sow ba she shesh peah
Asparagus officinalis

Fay Lyn He Does It of St. Xavier tells me that asparagus grows up along Soap Creek not far from our home on the Crow Reservation. I've never much cared for wild asparagus, but those who do talk on and on about it. If you decide to go after wild asparagus, you need to pick them at just the right time or the spears will be tough and stringy. Grandmother had no use for this particular plant food.

Camas Root: Basashbita upboop balusua
Camassia quamash

Growing up, we didn't pick all of the wild plants that we ate. One of my favorite treats doesn't even grow near here: camas roots, baked. They're from the west. Pretty Shield would trade something with the Piegan Indians when they came through with their roots. They had already baked the camas in the ground for four days, and they were delicious. The outside was black and a bit leathery—not really tough but rather chewy, kind of like a prune—and the whole thing had a wonderful licorice-like flavor. Pretty Shield would give them to us for snacks, and I used to steal away with as many as I could and eat them behind some tree.

Wild Greens

Once you start learning about edible plants, you start seeing them everywhere. Within a short walk from my house, I can find arrow-leaf balsamroot, stinging nettles, burdock, Indian lettuce, watercress,

A TASTE OF HERITAGE FOODS

and dandelions. In fields nearby grow lamb's quarters and pigweed. Some people consider all these plants to be weeds, but they are all edible greens. Some are tough and some are bitter, but you could eat any of them in a pinch, and I know some people who just love the taste of all of them.

Indian lettuce, miner's lettuce, dandelions, and lamb's quarters can all be eaten raw. If you want to eat arrow-leaf balsamroot, nettles, or burdock, you'll need to boil them, drain the water, and boil them again. That makes them a little less bitter and a little more tender, but those are some plants for which I would need to be really hungry before I spent much time picking. However, they are really good for you—lots of vitamins and minerals.

Indian Lettuce: Becashua ba luasua
Montia species
Miner's lettuce

Indian lettuce makes me feel good. I was very weary one day from tending to this and that, and wild lettuce was in abundance. I ate a handful and sat out on my deck. As I sat there, this wonderful feeling of well-being came over me, and lettuce has been my favorite relaxant ever since.

❧ Native American Salad

I discovered this modern adaptation for some favorite wild foods by trial and error.

4 cups Indian lettuce
1/2 cup wild carrots, diced
2 cups watercress
1/2 cup beef or buffalo tallow melted with 1/2 cup crushed wild turnips
Turnip bread, cubed and toasted (or other croutons)

Combine the Indian lettuce, wild carrots, and watercress and toss. Add the melted tallow with the crushed turnips. Toss gently and then add the turnip bread croutons.

Serves 4.

Dandelion: Ba oohba she lay

Taraxacum officinale

Despite dandelion's many medicinal uses, we mostly thought of dandelion as an extra little food when I was growing up. The leaves are very bitter. I like them that way, but I like the flowers best. The whole flower, fresh, has a bit of a sweet taste to it. When we were young we used to just go along and pick them and eat them. We were often hungry, and that snack probably satisfied some of our hunger.

Grandma always used to hold the flowers underneath our chins. If doing that reflects a yellow shade on your chin, it means you like butter. I don't know where she learned that, but she'd say it with a smile while looking at us. Of course it was true; we all liked butter.

✿ Dandelion Soup

This soup is a recipe from Bill's aunt Katy Birch.

4 potatoes, peeled and sliced
6 cups water
1 tablespoon salt (or less, according to taste)
¹/₂ pound dandelion leaves and stems, carefully rinsed
2 egg yolks
1 tablespoon margarine

Place the sliced potatoes in the water in a soup kettle. Add the salt and cook 15 minutes over medium heat. Then add the dandelion greens and simmer 15 minutes more. Beat together the egg yolks and margarine. Add to the soup and stir until well blended, about 1 minute. Serve hot with wild turnip bread or crackers, either broken up into the soup or eaten alongside separately.

Serves 4.

Wild Mushrooms

Mushrooms aren't a vegetable—they're fungi—but they are eaten like vegetables, so I'll talk about them here. Morels are the only wild mushrooms I've ever had any dealing with. They're very wrinkly little things, but they taste good, and nutritionists say they are good in a cancer-prevention diet. Morels are easiest to find after a fire.

After one fire they grew all over here in the Wolf Mountains. Someone collected a box of them and gave them to me, and I didn't know how to preserve them, so I gave them to everyone I knew who likes mushrooms. They were very tasty.

In general, however, I don't mess with mushrooms. There are too many dangerous ones. My grandma never did pick them or say much about them. The one exception was her telling us that if we stepped on toadstools, it would bring too much rain.

Garden Vegetables

My Father's Garden

Not everything we ate growing up was collected in the wild. Pretty Shield bought some food at the store, and many vegetables came straight from my father's garden.

Father, George Hogan, lived in Benteen, which wasn't really a town. Benteen Stockyards they called it, and it was on the edge of the Little Big Horn River. (Our home with Pretty Shield was a ways to the southwest.) He always had a garden, and in the summer when Pretty Shield was out collecting and drying ehe and berries and other wild things, he was growing and drying vegetables. He grew corn, peas, radishes, potatoes, beets, onions, carrots, pumpkins, and squash (mostly Hubbard squash).

He was also a very good cook. Father used dried peas in all sorts of things most people don't think of using them in. He'd tell us to go get as many peas as we could that were still on the vine. My sister would then go collect what carrots were still growing. Then he'd make a flour gravy and put it all together to make the best soup. He would always add herbs or spices.

I learned more about spices from my father than I did from Pretty Shield. I think I learned to use nutmeg from my father. He loved dumplings. Chicken and dumplings was one of his favorite foods. He always put a touch of nutmeg in the dumplings. Much later I remember a woman telling me, "That's very good. That's the secret of good dumplings."

✿ George Hogan's Chicken and Dumplings

    1 chicken
    Water
    1 teaspoon salt
    2 quarts chicken broth (see the recipe instructions)
    1 onion, minced
    2 cups all-purpose flour
    1 egg, slightly beaten
    2 teaspoons baking powder
    1/4 teaspoon salt
    1/8 teaspoon nutmeg

Clean and quarter the chicken. Place the quarters in a cast-iron roaster with boiling water to cover. Add the teaspoon of salt. Boil the chicken for at least one hour or until the meat comes easily off the bones. Separate the meat from the bones and set aside. Strain the broth, reserving 2 quarts.

In the roaster, simmer the minced onion in the reserved broth. Mix together the flour, egg, baking powder, salt, and nutmeg until the dough is light and fluffy. Drop the dough by rounded spoonfuls into the hot broth. Cover and cook for 10 to 15 minutes. Add the chicken pieces and serve.

Serves 8.

✿ My Father's Dried Peas and Carrot Gravy

At the end of the growing season, we gathered and shelled the dried peas in our garden, those that weren't picked fresh and green early in the summer. Father put the hard peas in water in a saucepan, covered them, and cooked them over medium heat for about an hour. Then he added chopped carrots and dried onions and continued cooking them for another 20 minutes. He thickened the mixture with flour (I'd recommend 3 heaping tablespoons of flour for every quart of liquid), seasoned it with salt and pepper, and served it for a simple but filling meal. If you'd like, add about 1/2 cup of canned milk (I like a little cream).

Squash: Coogooehsa

We'd dry the squash (Hubbard squash mostly), Grandma and I. We'd pick the huge vegetables off the vine in August and September, and later we'd cut them with sharp knives following a continuous circular pattern. A whole squash would become one long spiral of orange flesh with a blue-gray outer skin. You want to be sure the harvested squash sit a little while (maybe about two days off the vine) before you cut them this way or the piece will snap before you get to the end from being too crisp. You strip it in this continuous circle about 1-inch thick, and then you hang it over a tipi pole suspended on two posts, which are set in the shade. The squash is so heavy and thick that you wouldn't think it would dry the way it does, but it does. They say the spiral takes the wind and blows it through itself. If there's more than one squash hanging up, boy, it's a long tunnel for that wind to blow through! Being cut in a spiral dries it quicker and keeps the taste and the food value intact.

My editor thinks there is an art to cutting a squash all in one piece like that, but it didn't take me too long to learn it because Pretty Shield would make me feel the texture of the squash before I started. I was good at cutting squashes for drying. After I cut the squash, the seeds would nearly all fall out, and I would shake out the rest. Pretty Shield never ate the seeds. In fact, they were not used for any cooking at all as I remember.

We used the dried squash in stews. The Crows liked to stew those long circular pieces still whole, but you can cut them into strips three or four inches long. We would always cook it with the skin on.

ᏚᎢ Squash and Onion

My favorite traditional way to cook squash is with onions. Whole onions with the skin left on baked with pieces of squash give it a nice color; they give it kind of a red look. Just bake the squash and onions together, take them out of the oven, and if you like onions, you can eat them, or if you don't want the onion, you can eat just the squash and the cooking liquid. I put a little sugar with it myself because I have a sweet tooth. We use squash from our garden, but they can be purchased at the grocery store too.

1/2 Hubbard squash or 2 winter squash, sliced 1 inch thick
Water
Brown sugar
1 yellow onion, washed but not peeled

Place the winter squash slices in a roasting pan with enough water in the bottom to prevent scorching. Sprinkle the squash slices with brown sugar and place the unpeeled onion in between the squash. Bake covered in a medium oven until tender. Remove the onion (its nutrients are now in the juice), or just remove the onion skin and eat the onion along with the squash. The pan juice will appear red, which is my favorite part of the whole dish. You might serve the squash along with jerky and rice soup.

Serves 10 to 12 people.

Fruits

Nature provides fruit all through the summer in Crow country, from the first juneberries, which ripen at the very beginning of July here in Montana, to the buffaloberries, which ripen not until after the first frost. In the valley along the creeks we find chokecherries, plums, and buffaloberries. A bit higher up we find juneberries and elderberries. Up in the mountains grow raspberries, hawthorns, and strawberries. Further west in Montana are dark, juicy huckleberries. Out on the plains we can find cactus fruits, for something a little different. All these traditional wild fruits are easily adapted into modern recipes. They are easy to identify and easy to preserve. They provide important nutrients and taste great.

A TASTE OF HERITAGE FOODS

Different fruits work well in different recipes. If you don't have the fruit one recipe calls for, feel free to experiment with others that you have on hand. I've listed some favorites to help guide you. My favorite fruit to eat straight from the plant would have to be juneberries. After those, I like the red berries—raspberries and strawberries—and then plums and chokecherries. Juneberries make the best pie I think, but men always seem to prefer huckleberry or blueberry pie. Buffaloberries make the best jelly, and chokecherries are the easiest to dry. For making traditional pemmican, chokecherries are the tastiest, but juneberries work too.

Juneberry: Baáchuuawuuleete
Amelanchier alnifolia
Serviceberry, Sarviceberry, Saskatoon, Shad Bush

Of all the berries around here, when we were growing up we liked juneberries the best. We liked them best because they were smooth in the mouth. They didn't have so much grit to them, the way that some of the other wild berries did. We used to like to eat juneberries plain. We also made pudding out of them. We made pemmican too. We even took the juice and washed our eyes out with it.

We'd go up to the mountains in early July and if we came home with a big galvanized washtub almost full, Pretty Shield was satisfied. (Even though the English name is "juneberry," they are rarely ripe in June around here. It seems we always pick juneberries in July.) We dried them and later on people froze them, but Pretty Shield was never much for freezing. She dried everything. Juneberries can be dried whole. I have some dried juneberries that I show at presentations that are more than thirty years old. If I soaked them and then cooked them, they would still taste like juneberries. They wouldn't be as good as fresh, of course, but they would still be edible. Dried juneberries keep real well.

Like a plum or chokecherry, a juneberry is a shrub or small tree that grows near creeks in the foothills and up into the mountains. Also like plums and chokecherries, they have pretty white blossoms in the spring. Unlike plums or cherries, though, juneberries do not have pits. The Crow name is *baáchuuawuuleete* (and sounds like "ba zha a woo le de"), which means "berry without big seeds." Juneberries do have seeds, but unlike those of the other fruits, they are so small that you don't notice them. Berry pudding, called *balapia*, is usually made from juneberries mixed with other berries and then sweetened and thickened. We eat it at every celebration.

Juneberry juice is also used for a purple dye. The juice is very strong. Its color won't wash out. Juneberries also settle the stomach and have a calming effect, and you can read about their benefits for the eyes in the medicinal plants chapter. Still, we generally think of juneberries as just a tasty food.

⁕ Balapia: Berry Pudding

This traditional dessert is served at all special occasions. I keep frozen berries on hand year-round to make this pudding, since a feast or celebration wouldn't be complete without it. This recipe can be easily doubled for large groups, and the pudding tastes great by itself or over ice cream for a special treat. Juneberries and raspberries are most commonly used in the pudding, but different combinations of berries all taste good.

1 quart juneberries
Water
Sugar to taste
3 heaping tablespoons cornstarch or 4 tablespoons wild turnip flour
1 teaspoon vanilla extract (optional)
1 cup raspberries (optional)

Place the juneberries in a pot and cover with water to about 2 inches above the berries. Cook until the berries are plump. Add sugar according to your taste and the sweetness of the berries. For every quart of liquid in the pot measure in 3 tablespoons of cornstarch or 4 tablespoons of turnip flour. Cook until the thickener dissolves and the mixture begins to thicken, about ten more minutes. Add vanilla and raspberries, if desired. It's best when served warm.

≈ Juneberry Pie

While pies are not a traditional food among Indian people, the ingredients around here are perfect for them. Juneberry sauce or pudding has been eaten for a long, long time, and when we had bread we would eat them with bread. It's just another step to go from berry sauce and bread to a pie.

I happened to be making this juneberry pie when Pascale LeDraoulec, a food writer, called me up out of the blue. She stopped by, watched me bake a pie, and wrote about it in her book American Pie.

1 cup water
2 cups ripe juneberries
$2/3$ cup sugar
3 tablespoons cornstarch
1 teaspoon vanilla extract
2 tablespoons butter (or vegetable shortening or margarine)
Basic pie crust for a two-crust pie, unbaked (recipe follows)

In a saucepan heat the cup of water to a simmer and then add the berries, sugar, cornstarch, and vanilla. Cook while stirring constantly. Then let the mixture cool. Pour it into the pie shell. Spread pieces of butter over the sauce. Cover with a top crust. Bake at 350 degrees until the crust is nice and brown, about 35 minutes.

≈ Basic Pie Crust for a Two-crust Pie

2 cups all-purpose flour
1 teaspoon salt
2 teaspoons sugar
1/3 cup vegetable oil, shortening, or butter
6 to 8 tablespoons cold water
1 egg yolk (optional; save the white to brush on top)

Mix together the flour, salt, and sugar. Crumble the oil in with your fingers or cut in the shortening or butter with a pastry blender until the crumbs are the size of small peas. Add the egg yolk (which is optional, but it seems to make the dough easier to work with) and enough cold water to hold the dough together. Divide the dough in half. Place one half of the dough on a floured board and roll it out until it's evenly about $1/4$-inch thick and large enough to fill a 9-inch pie plate.

Roll out the second portion of the dough and reserve it for the top of the pie. Prick vent holes in the top crust after assembling the pie. I like to crimp the two crusts together with my thumb and forefinger to make a wavy edge and cut three small slits in four places on the top to let the steam out. A beaten egg white brushed on the top crust will give the whole pie a nice golden glaze.

❧ Juneberry Chiffon Pie

1 cup juneberries
1 1/4 cups water, divided
4 eggs, yolks and whites separated
1/2 cup sugar, divided
1 tablespoon unflavored gelatin
1 teaspoon vanilla
1 baked piecrust (graham cracker is best)
Whipped cream for topping

Boil the juneberries in 1 cup of water. Cook for 20 minutes. Strain the berries through a sieve and set aside.

Beat the 4 egg yolks lightly. Stir in 1/4 cup of sugar. Place the egg yolks and sugar in the top of a double boiler. Stir constantly until the mixture thickens and then add the strained berries.

Soften the tablespoon of gelatin in 1/4 cup of cold water and add to the custard mixture in the double boiler. Cook, stirring, until the gelatin dissolves. Remove the pan from the heat, add the vanilla, and cool.

Beat the 4 egg whites until stiff and then add the second 1/4 cup of sugar a little at a time. Continue beating until completely mixed.

Take the cooled pudding and fold it a little at a time into the beaten egg whites. Pour the mixture into the prepared piecrust. Top with whipped cream.

❧ Juneberry Cake with Orange

  1 pint juneberries
  1 1/2 cups water
  1 3/4 cups all-purpose flour, sifted
  1/4 teaspoon salt
  6 eggs, separated
  1 1/2 cups sugar, divided
  6 tablespoons orange juice
  1 teaspoon grated orange peel
  Confectioner's sugar

Cook the juneberries in the water for about 15 minutes and then set aside. In a mixing bowl, sift together the flour and salt. In another bowl, beat the egg whites until foamy. Gradually add 1/2 cup of the sugar, about 2 tablespoons at a time, beating well after each addition. Continue beating until stiff peaks form and then set aside. Preheat the oven to 350 degrees. In a small bowl, beat the egg yolks until they are thick and lemon colored. Gradually beat in the remaining 1 cup of sugar until smooth. Add the flour and salt mixture while beating on a slow speed, alternating with adding the orange juice and juneberries. Stop beating and gently fold in the egg whites and orange peel. Pour the batter into a greased and floured 9 x 5 x 2 inch cake pan and bake for 35 minutes, or until golden brown. Cool and sprinkle with confectioner's sugar.

🍃 Juneberry Marmalade

   2 cups juneberries
   2 cups sugar
   1 ¹/₂ cups water
   1 envelope or bottle pectin
   Grated peel of ¹/₂ lemon
   Grated peel of ¹/₂ orange

   Cook the juneberries and sugar in the water over low heat until the berries are soft and cooked. Remove from the heat and whirl in a blender. Add the pectin, following the manufacturer's directions, and the grated citrus peels. Cook an additional 5 minutes. Pour into sterilized jars with lids and seal following canning instructions or use immediately. Enjoy on homemade bread or toast.

   Makes about 4 half-pint jars of marmalade.

Raspberries: Baaxuaga
Rubus species

Wild raspberries, *baaxuaga*, don't grow in the Little Big Horn Valley, so we'd travel once a year to pick them from the *chateish*, the Wolf Mountains. One lady whom we traveled with, going up there to camp, would take along her open canner and jars. She had a big family, and they needed all the food they could put away for the winter. She brought her canning supplies to save the raspberries because after we picked them, they just seemed to settle themselves down, crush themselves, no matter what sort of container we would put them into. If you pick half a kettle of raspberries one day, the next morning the kettle will be only a quarter full. That's what this woman didn't like. To prevent that, she'd take along her canner and everything and use it right on an open fire. She'd put her jars of raspberries in the canner and seal them right there and put them in the boxes to bring home. The fresh raspberries didn't have a chance to settle down to nothing when she did that.

   Grandma didn't take her canning things to the mountains like that. She didn't dry the raspberries or freeze them either. We just ate them.

We threw them in our mouths and ate them. We'd eat them while we were picking them and then get them home and eat some more. Those raspberries would soon be all eaten up.

Gooseberries and Currants: Be ga ge ta
Ribes species

Gooseberries are longevity berries to me. Older Assiniboine women say gooseberries keep you from being too tired. In other words, gooseberries keep you young. They give you stamina, energy, and build you right up so you can continue to go on every day. If you eat a lot of gooseberries and currants, you can achieve longevity.

Bill's folks used to eat gooseberries a lot (the word is *win check gon sa* in Assiniboine), and they wouldn't clean them off or anything. They'd just cook them still with their little tails. (Gooseberries have a small spiny point on the bottom of the berry.)

Bill once said, "There are sticks in here."

His mother, Blue Robe, answered, "Oh just eat it, sticks and all."

Currants and gooseberries can be used in almost all of the same ways. Whichever type you pick, you need to get out there and pick them as soon as they are ripe; otherwise they just dry up on the vine. They don't all ripen at the same time either: some are ready in late June and others in July. You need to keep watching them and get them just when they are purple and ripe. Like all the other berries, you can dry them if you want to, and currants and gooseberries both make good sauces.

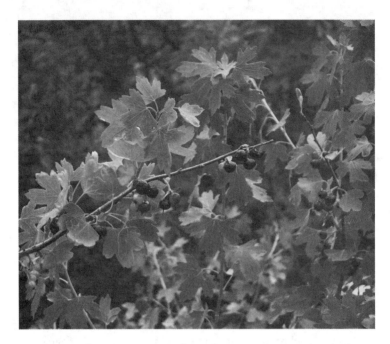

Currants

❧ Gooseberry Pudding

If you want a more authentic Assiniboine longevity food, make this pudding, "sticks and all." Bob and James Krumm included my gooseberry pudding recipe in The Pacific Northwest Berry Book, *but of course they left out the little twigs.*

3 tablespoons cornstarch
1 cup water
1 quart gooseberries
2 cups sugar

In a saucepan, dissolve the cornstarch in the water. Add the gooseberries and sugar and cook until the mixture is thickened. Serve warm, as is.

Serves 8.

A TASTE OF HERITAGE FOODS

Elderberry: Balawoolatebagua
Sambucus racemosa
Hollowwood berry

Balawoolatebagua, "hollow wood berries"—that's the name we give to elderberries. Both the flowers and fruits of this shrubby elderbush are edible, but watch out! Bears like them too! Three years back, a black bear pawed down an elderberry bush right behind our house. He mauled it until there was almost nothing left, but it came back and has grown strong since then. Lisa, my editor, was telling one of her friends about the wildlife here and said, "A bear mauled an elder right behind the house." Lisa couldn't figure out why her friend was so shocked. Of course, she was talking about an elderberry bush, and her friend was thinking a bear had eaten an old Indian right on our back step.

Elderberries make good pies. Men especially like to eat elderberry pie, right up there with blueberry and huckleberry pies. Women like it too, but the men always request it. The dark purple jelly from elderberries is also real tasty. Be careful though. The juice from elderberries stains. That's good when you are making dye but not so good if you get it on your white clothes while you are making jelly.

If you can't wait for the elderberries, you can eat the blossoms. I cut up the lacy flowerheads—which can be seven or eight inches in diameter—into small sizes and mix them in with my hotcake batter. We learned about using these blossoms from some pioneer friends. We kind of followed likewise when we saw them putting them in their batter. The blossoms extend the number of hotcakes you can make. And they are very good—very good and nutritious.

Elderberry branches were always used for peashooters. Some kids that were musical tried to use them for flutes, but I don't think they work as well for that as the hardwoods.

The dark (black) elderberries are the good ones. The species that produces red berries is poisonous, and some say that even eating raw too many of the good black ones will make you sick to your stomach. I've also read that the hollow stems of the elderberry shouldn't

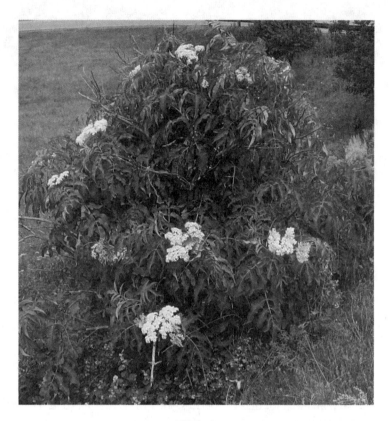

Elderbush

be used as peashooters or whistles because of poisonous compounds in the plants, but I have never heard of any Crow child having problems with this.

Chokecherry: Baju dala
Prunus virginiana

Chokecherries are one of the most useful plants that grow around here. The small tree provides food, a medicine, and good wood, all in one. Some boys save the pits and shoot them through hollow elderberry stems, using them as peashooters, so I guess chokecherry seeds can be used as toys too.

Traditional Chokecherry Foods

As kids, we would ride our horses bareback out to where the choke-cherries grow, eat a few of them right there from the bushes, and bring the rest back to Pretty Shield in big baskets.

My grandmother crushed the chokecherries between rocks. She used her pestle and her rock platform, and she would absolutely mash those seeds and everything all together. She and her friends would form the cherry mash into little patties after they had crushed the fruit and would place them on a tarp. They placed the patties about half a foot apart to dry.

Sometimes they'd squeeze the chokecherry mash through their hands so that it formed a shape like a railroad spike. They would dry the spikes just as they would the patties. I used to like dried cherries that way because I could hold the spikes and eat them easier than I could the flat patties.

To make the mash dry evenly, we'd turn the chokecherry patties often. When we turned them, the underside would look very pink, so then we knew by comparison that the top had dried. Always we tried to do our drying in the shade. I know that some say to dry fruit in the sun, but food dried in the shade was what we liked. My grandmother thought the taste stayed within the substance when it was dried in the shade, away from direct sunlight.

Once dried, we used the crushed chokecherries as a snack. We would sweeten the chokecherry crush with a little sugar in a bowl. We stuck bread in there and scooped it out and ate it that way. We also mixed crushed chokecherries with our jerky and grease to make pemmican. When we made pemmican, we kept a little chokecherry juice so we could warm the fat in it. The Crow Indian women really liked dried cherries ground fine and put in with the pemmican, and that's what they say real pemmican is: crushed chokecherries and kidney tallow mixed with pulverized dry meat. Fat and the moist chokecherries held the mixture together.

If they weren't dried, cherries were fixed in a sauce. They boiled them, and they thickened the sauce, either with turnip flour or regu-

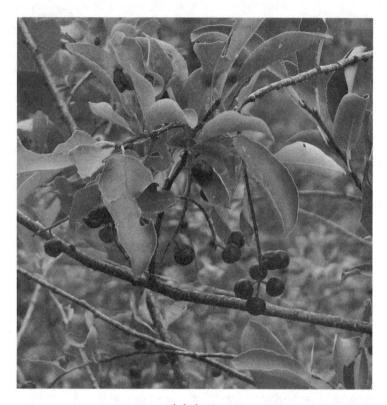

Chokecherries

lar flour or cornstarch, and they put sugar in it. I put a little almond flavoring in it today. Simmer the cherries in a kettle for about 20 minutes. The Crows used to eat chokecherries that way and spit out the seeds. That's the way I've seen them eat it as a sauce.

Up at Fort Belknap, Bill's aunt used to grind up chokecherries real fine, and then she'd put tallow with the cherry meal that resulted. She'd melt the grease first, and then she'd mix it with the ground chokecherries and put it on her bread. The mixture made what was a jam to her. She liked it that way, but I don't especially care for it myself.

A TASTE OF HERITAGE FOODS

Pretty Shield protected us from eating too much of anything with chokecherries in it. Cherries had a binding effect, and we would suffer from plugged-up bowels if we ate too much. My grandmother allowed us to eat about a cup, and that was all. We didn't ask for any more because we didn't like what happened when we did eat too many cherries.

Bill thinks the seeds are a little bit too hard for a person.

Modern Chokecherry Foods

The Indians learned from the agriculture workers that chokecherry syrup made from chokecherry juice is very good as a flavoring. They put a little sugar in the chokecherry juice and put it on hotcakes and bread. I think it's even better over ice cream. Take chokecherry syrup, heat it a little bit, and pour it over ice cream. It makes a great sundae. That's what I have been doing lately. It tastes great.

Chokecherries also make a very good jelly. I don't care too much for chokecherry jam, but I like the clear jelly very well. Cook and process chokecherries the same way you would crabapples. After cooking them, squeeze them through a cloth to get only the juice.

﹐ Chokecherry Sauce

I think the almond flavoring really adds something to this simple sauce, but of course you can leave it out or try it with vanilla extract instead. Use chokecherry sauce on biscuits, ice cream, or even over crepes, if you want to be gourmet. It also goes well with duck and other wild fowl.

1 quart chokecherries
4 tablespoons sugar
1 teaspoon almond extract

Wash and drain the chokecherries. Grind the cherries whole in a strong food processor. Pour the processed cherries through a sieve or strainer and catch the fruit in a saucepan. Add the sugar and almond extract and simmer for 15 minutes. Remove from the heat and cool slightly before serving.

❧ Chokecherry Cake

    2 cups all-purpose flour, sifted

    2 cups sugar

    1 teaspoon baking soda

    1 teaspoon salt

    $^1/_2$ teaspoon baking powder

    $^3/_4$ cup water

    $^3/_4$ cup milk

    $^1/_2$ cup shortening, melted

    2 eggs, slightly beaten

    1 teaspoon almond extract

    1 cup crushed chokecherries

Mix together the flour, sugar, baking soda, salt, and baking powder with a wire whip. Add the water and milk along with the melted shortening and eggs and combine. Add the almond extract, and lastly add the crushed cherries. Mix well by hand. Pour the batter into a greased and floured angel food cake pan. Bake for 45 minutes at 350 degrees F.

Huckleberries: Kapi:lia:zde

Vaccinium species

Huckleberries don't grow around Ft. Smith, Montana, where I live now, but in the mountains of northwestern Montana, they grow all over the place. It seems that men and bears can't get enough of them. Bill's favorite fruit is huckleberry, either raw or in pie.

Huckleberry Pie

Huckleberries are tarter than many other wild berries. You may wish to omit the lemon juice. If you can't find huckleberries, store-bought blueberries make a tasty pie as well.

Like most other Crow women of my generation, I learned about the art of pie baking in home economics class. I learned home economics at the Flandreau Boarding School in South Dakota.

This is Bill's favorite pie.

4 cups huckleberries
1 cup sugar
6 tablespoons cornstarch
²/₃ cup water, approximately
1 tablespoon lemon juice
2 tablespoons butter
Basic pie crust for a two-crust pie (see recipe in juneberry section)

Cook the huckleberries for about 20 minutes over medium heat with the sugar. Mix the cornstarch with a small amount of water (just enough to wet the cornstarch, so it does not make lumps). Add the cornstarch mixture to the berries along with the lemon juice and butter. Cook, stirring constantly, until the mixture thickens. Remove from the heat.

Bake an unfilled bottom crust in a 350-degree oven until it is half done, about five minutes. (This step keeps the crust from becoming soggy.)

Pour the berry filling into the half-baked crust. Roll out the other half of the dough. Place the dough on top of the pie, dab with butter, and continue baking until golden brown, about 40 minutes.

❧ Blackberry Pie

When Bill and I lived in Oregon, we picked a lot of wild blackberries. They don't grow in Crow territory, but they sure are abundant over in the Pacific Northwest. If you don't have access to wild blackberries, buy some at your store or substitute raspberries.

Basic pie crust for a single-crust pie
1 egg white, lightly whipped
3 cups blackberries
1/2 cup brown sugar
1 tablespoon flour
1 cup sour cream

Line a pie plate with the pie-crust pastry. Brush it all over with the whipped egg white for firmness. Fill the pie with blackberries. In a bowl, combine the brown sugar, flour, and sour cream. Cover the berries with this mixture. Bake at 450 degrees for 10 minutes. Reduce the oven temperature to 350 degrees and bake for 40 minutes more. Serve warm.

Grapes: Dax bee chay ish ta shay
Vitus species
Slick Bears' Eyes

Fresh wild grapes. Oh, they are good. I love to eat them fresh, just as they are. I used to eat so many of them; I ate them until my mouth itched. I ate them until it itched and itched and itched. Then it would hurt so much that I would have to quit eating altogether.

The Crows call wild grapes "slick bears' eyes," *dax bee chay ish ta shay*. You can just see those wild grapes down by the creek shining at you like bears' eyes in the trees. Grandma crushed the grapes, the whole cluster—berries, little stems, and all—and dried them in little patties. We ate them in pudding too, a pudding sauce. Now we make syrup out of grapes and keep the juice. We have lots of juice. Of course you can also make jellies and jams.

Besides the regular wild grapes, which grow on grapevines running through the trees, you can also find the Oregon grape (Mahonia *repens*) up in the mountains. While I have never seen many fruits on one of those little plants, you can eat the grapes right off of them, and they do taste like flavorful little grapes.

ᔥ Dried Grape Berries

> Pick wild grapes when they're ripe, which is usually in the middle of summer. Wash and crush them with the stems and seeds included. Place on a tarp by tablespoonfuls, just here and there on the tarp. Smooth them over a little to form round patties. Let them dry in the air, preferably in the shade on a sunny day. After drying we stored them in cotton bags made just for this purpose.

Grapes were eaten to enjoy as is, or they were sauced. Later we would take the grape patties and put them in a saucepan with just enough water to cover them. We'd simmer them about twenty minutes, add a little sugar if we wanted them sweeter, and then eat them hot or cold.

American Indians also knew the potential grapes had in healing. For more about their medicinal value, see chapter 6.

Kinnikinnick: Obeezia

Arctostaphylos uva-ursi

Bearberry

Up on Bill's reservation (Fort Belknap), his mother and aunts and everyone would all get together, and they would take a wagon with all their canning supplies right on it and go into the hills for a few days to pick and preserve the kinnikinnick berries. They would camp in the hills, and they would have fiddle dances at night and just have a great time. Right there they would make and preserve this apple butter–like paste with the berries. They never did this when I was around, and they haven't done it for a long time now. But I always listen to these stories, and Bill has told me that he went along once when he was young.

Blue Robe, Bill's mother, and his aunts made the kinnikinnick butter. They called it *larb*. It tastes great, and from the stories it always sounds like they had a great time when they were out collecting the berries.

Kinnikinnick berries, bearberries, can be eaten raw, but they are awfully bitter. They're not sweet enough for me. Bill's family always added sweetener when they made the butter.

❧ Bearberry Butter

Bearberries
Water
Sugar
Pectin

Pick bearberries. Place them in a large saucepan with enough water to cover. Cook until the berries open up, and then strain them through a berry sieve. Throw the seeds away. Add sugar to sweeten as you like. Place the berries and sugar back in the saucepan and cook. Use 1 package of pectin to about 6 quarts of berry pulp (follow the directions on the packet of pectin). Put the mixture into hot, sterilized pint jars. Seal and sterilize. Spread on bread like apple butter.

Makes about 8 pints.

Wild Plum: Buluhpe
Prunus americana

Wild plums grow on shrubby little trees alongside creeks. They are beautiful when they bloom in May, and the fruit can be picked in August. As for most wild fruits, you really need to watch them as they are ripening to make sure you get them before the birds and animals do. The birds and animals really seem to know the very moment the fruits become ripe.

My grandma, Pretty Shield, said the moon ripens the plums. She went more by the moon and less by the sun. She says the moon has a lot to do with water, and the moisture in the plum is pulled apart by the moon. As the moon pulls the plums apart, they ripen easily.

With grandma we boiled the plums, pitted them and we took the juice and after we did that we cooled it off and we took the seeds out of them. We'd take the pulp and the juice and make a sauce, a plum sauce. That's good but I always thought you needed a bit more sugar to make me really chew the skin. My grandmother used to take the plums, smush them together into little piles and dry them that way, or just scatter them and dry them. They were not hard to prepare.

Today I put pitted plums in my mixer, pulp and all, blend them up, cook them down, and then put my spices to them. I call it Indian Ketchup because I make it out of the wild stuff, and it's sort of spicy and modern. It's really good on buffalo jerky and other meat.

ᚚ Indian Ketchup

This recipe can be doubled, and the resulting sauce can be canned and stored for future use.

2 $^1/_2$ quarts wild plums
1 cup water
$^1/_2$ teaspoon baking soda
2 pounds sugar
1 cup apple cider vinegar
1 $^1/_4$ teaspoons cloves
$^3/_4$ teaspoon cinnamon
1 $^1/_2$ teaspoon allspice

Boil the plums in the water with the baking soda. Bring them to a rolling boil. When they're cooked, strain the plums through a cloth or sieve. Return the pulp and juice to the stove and heat. Add the sugar, vinegar, cloves, cinnamon, and allspice and simmer until thickened.

ᶘ Plum Good Indian Pudding

  1 quart wild plum juice
  1 teaspoon rum extract
  1 cup yellow cornmeal
  2 tablespoons butter, melted
  1/2 cup molasses
  1 teaspoon salt
  2 eggs

Heat the plum juice and rum extract in a saucepan and then pour it over the cornmeal in the top of a double boiler. Stir constantly. Cook the mixture over hot water for 20 minutes. Heat the oven to 350 degrees. Combine the melted butter, molasses, and salt and stir into the cornmeal mixture. Beat the eggs well and add to the cornmeal. Pour this mixture into a greased 5 x 8 x 2 inch baking dish. Place the baking dish in a larger pan half filled with water and bake for 1 hour. Serve warm with whipped cream or ice cream, if desired.

ᶘ Plum Bread

Because we had few cooking utensils and pans when I was growing up, it was important to learn to make do with what we did have. We were taught by agricultural extension agents to save certain cans and use them for baking pans. This recipe uses coffee cans, but you can bake the bread in regular loaf pans, if you prefer.

  1 1/2 cups yellow cornmeal
  2 cups all-purpose flour
  2 1/2 teaspoons baking soda
  1 teaspoon salt
  1 1/3 cups buttermilk
  3/4 cups dark molasses
  1 cup plums
  Boiling water

Into a large bowl, sift together the cornmeal, flour, baking soda, and salt. In a small bowl, combine the buttermilk and molasses. Mix the liquid ingredients into the dry ingredients. Stir in the plums. Spoon the batter into two well-greased one-pound coffee cans, filling them two-thirds full. Tie pieces of heavy foil over the tops of the cans. Place the cans in a large pan containing water and cover the pan with heavy foil. Steam for 2 ½ to 3 hours at 350 degrees, adding more boiling water as needed. Test for doneness with a table knife. Cool on a rack when the knife comes out clean.

Serves 10.

✿ Spicy Dried Plum Cake

Prunes made from commercial plums were a common food that the government distributed to the Crow people. Most people can eat only so many prunes straight out of the bag, so they started asking me what else they could do with them. I found a good spice cake recipe and added prunes to it. The result is moist and tasty, and it has become a tradition for special occasions in my family.

If you want to give this cake more of a "wild" flavor, you could substitute dried wild plums for the prunes, leave out the cloves, and add a teaspoon of rum. I like cloves better, but if rum is preferred, use 1 teaspoon and add it when you put in the oil and eggs.

2 cups water
2 cups pitted prunes
4 cups all-purpose flour
3 cups sugar
2 ½ teaspoons baking soda
2 teaspoons salt
2 teaspoons cinnamon
2 teaspoons nutmeg
2 teaspoons cloves
1 cup vegetable oil
6 eggs

Grease and flour 2 Bundt cake pans. Set the oven at 350 degrees. Mix together all the ingredients. Pour the batter evenly divided into the two cake pans and bake for 45 minutes to 1 hour.

Hawthorns: Beelee chi sha yeah
Crataegus species

The fruits of the hawthorn trees, which look like little crab apples, can be used both as food and medicine. You can read about the way these special fruits were harvested with care and prayer in chapter 6. Here, I offer some simple recipes for those just wanting a taste of this unusual fruit. Of course if a person is taking heart medication prescribed by a doctor, the doctor's approval is necessary to use hawthorn berry in any form.

❧ Hawthorn Berry Sauce

Like apples and most other wild fruits, hawthorn fruits vary greatly as to how sweet they are. Add only a little sugar at a time until the sauce reaches the sweetness you desire.

> 3 pounds hawthorn berries
> Water
> Sugar to taste
> Cinnamon to taste (about 1 1/2 teaspoons)

Cook the berries in a large stainless-steel pot with just enough water to cover them for about 1 hour or until they are soft. Carefully strain the berries through a sieve. Sweeten to taste and then add cinnamon to taste. Fill clean, sterilized pint jars, seal, sterilize, and store.

Cactuses: Bigeelia

Prickly Pear: Bitchgalee ba a ba lee gish sha
Opuntia species

Pincushion Cactus: Bitchgalee bajua
Coryphantha species

Two kinds of cactus grow in Crow country. Prickly pears are good to eat, once you remove the spines. Chopping them or peeling them like a pear both work for getting at the edible pulp inside.

Less common but better to eat are the little pincushion cactuses. When I was just married, we had a lot of those up at my husband's place. They have sweet red berries in the crown of each section that we call cactus berries. They are so sweet to eat. Better still are the green fig-sized pieces from the middle of the cactus. Eaten fresh they are just wonderful. They are a little harder than the cactus berries. The stickers are all on the head of the cactus, but the figlike part in the middle is completely smooth.

My son, Billy, some thirteen years later, harvested cactus for profit. When we were living in Harlem, Montana, and he was in about the sixth grade, he would go out back and fill his pockets with those little cactus parts (after he pulled out the small clusters of prickles with tweezers, of course). He would sell these to his friends. He would sell them for five cents a piece, mind you. His friends would all buy them from him, and he would have all the movie and popcorn money he wanted.

Roses: Bijaba
Rosa species

The wild roses brightening the hillsides of Crow country with their cheerful pink flowers have several edible parts: shoots, flowers, and fruits.

Once cleaned and peeled, the very young shoots of rosebushes are fresh, tasty, and wonderfully crunchy. Rose petals, too, are good to eat. They add a lot to a salad and taste especially good with cucumbers.

The fruits of the wild rose, called rose hips, are edible. Full of vitamin C, the fruits can be eaten fresh, if you watch out for all the seeds. Assiniboine kids know them as "itchberry" because they make your bottom itch if you eat too many of them fresh. I don't recommend eating many with the seeds intact.

Rose hips traditionally were crushed, seeded, and mixed with tallow to be put away for winter use. Grandmother Pretty Shield would find a nice hole about two to three feet deep by the bank of a river, put cool rocks in it, put the tallow and rose hips in, and cover it with more rocks. She'd leave it stored away in that cool place for winter use.

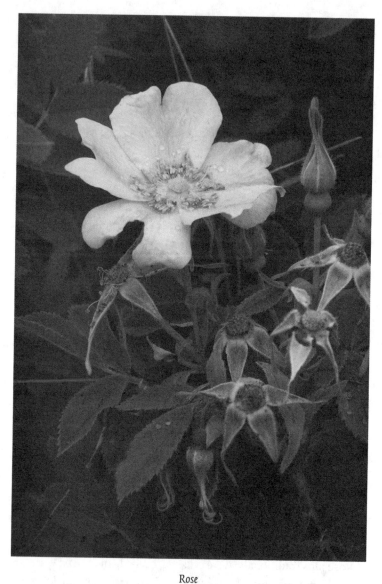

Rose

A TASTE OF HERITAGE FOODS

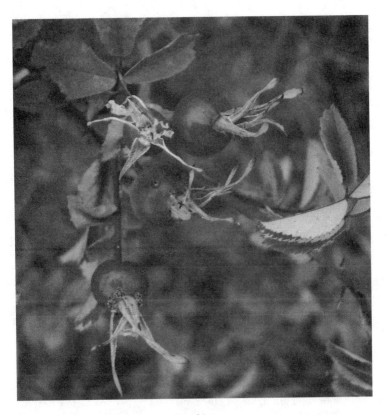

Rose hips

Meanwhile, in summer the mixture was eaten any time as a kind of summer pemmican.

Different types of roses have different amounts of seeds, pulp, and hairs on the little fruits. You might need to press the cooked hips through a sieve or even cheesecloth depending on how seedy they are and how smooth you want your sauce. The roses in your yard might work great for these recipes, but remember not to use them if you have been spraying the plants with pesticides.

❧ Rose Hip Sauce for Meat

This modern rose hip sauce is an excellent addition to a meal of roasted or grilled venison.

2 cups rose hips, seeded
1 1/2 cups water
1/2 cup sugar
3 tablespoons cornstarch
1/2 cup white wine (optional)

Simmer the rose hips in the water for 1 hour. Add the sugar and cook for 5 more minutes. Add the cornstarch and continue simmering for 3 minutes, stirring constantly. Add the white wine just before serving, if desired.

❧ Sweet Rose Hip Sauce

Pour this sauce over ice cream for a delicious, different taste.

2 cups rose hips, seeded
2 cups water
1/4 cup honey
1/2 cup wild turnip flour (or substitute 2 tablespoons cornstarch)

Cook the rose hips in the water until soft (about 20 minutes). Add the honey and turnip flour to the remaining pulp. Cook on low heat for another 20 minutes, stirring constantly. Remove from the heat and serve.

A TASTE OF HERITAGE FOODS

Buffaloberry: Baishhesha
Sheperdia canadensis
Bullberry

Long ago, mountain men went out trapping and looking for gold, coming back to camp only once a year. When they returned each year, the women would serve them buffalo with a sauce made out of "buffalo berries" because they tasted great together. The mountain men came to expect this delicious meal.

One year they arrived back at camp, but there was no sauce made of buffalo berries for the meat. They really wanted some, but they could not communicate to the women what they were talking about. Finally they started signing. First they made a little horn and scratched the earth, pretending to be a bull buffalo, and then they pointed to the meat: "this buffalo." The women, of course, understood that. It was just the *sauce* thing they couldn't figure out. After acting out many cooking motions and pretending to roll little berries between their fingers and pinching their cheeks to make them red, the men were finally able to explain what they wanted. The Indian women figured out what the mountain men were talking about, and although they didn't have any crushed buffalo berries that year, they got on the "moccasin telegraph" and somebody down the way brought some over.

Since then the English word has always been buffaloberry, or bullberry, because the mountain men wanted them on their buffalo meat—not because the buffalo eat the berries. The Crow word is completely different, *ba ish he sha*, meaning "red face," and it is so named because the pungency of the berry gives the eater a red face. More recently, the Crow language has changed, and the way the younger generation says it, *ba lish he sha*, it sounds like "red jerky."

Those are the stories of all the names of the buffaloberry, a pungent little red berry, the last one of the season. Big stands of it grow on bushes here along the Big Horn River. The small trees have beautiful silver leaves and these tempting-looking red berries. But pick a red buffaloberry too soon, and you will be in for a shock. They are very tart before the first frost. After the first frost, they are much easier to pick, and they taste much sweeter. You just have to wait.

Buffaloberry sauce on buffalo meat is the traditional way to eat this food, and boy is that a good combination. Just cook the berries with sugar and a little flour or cornstarch. You can dry them too. My grandmother used to crush them, and then every so often she would place them on the spread-out tarp. She would dry them that way, in the shade on a sunny day. Then she put them away in sacks, just as she stored the chokecherries.

Buffaloberries also make excellent jelly. It is bright red and just the right combination of tart and sweet. Just fix the jam as you would for any other berry. These berries make very good jelly and very good jam.

Harvest

If you like your berries real sharp, you can pick buffaloberries any time, but, as I said before, they come off the twig easier after the first frost, and they are also much sweeter. Picking them involves at least two people. First place a tarp underneath the plant. Then one person pulls down a branch and holds it down. The other person pounds on the branch with a stick. All the berries fall onto the tarp. Then you gather up the edges of the tarp and pour the berries into your buckets. You clean the berries afterward.

You never clean buffaloberries in your house. They are dirtier than other berries and have little bugs all over them. Somehow the berry is not harmed by the bugs, but you have to watch out that you don't bring them into the house. To clean the berries, I used to put them in water outside, next to the house. I would bring my berries and put them in a tub of water and take out all the leaves and twigs floating on it and throw them away. But I wouldn't throw them away right next to the house because there would be stickers, worms, and earwigs, and we didn't want them to grow and multiply around the house. So we put all the floating stuff into a container, put a lid on it so the insects wouldn't get out, and threw it away with the garbage going to the dump.

A TASTE OF HERITAGE FOODS

❧ Buffaloberry Meat Sauce

Crush buffaloberries until they look like raw hamburger. Serve on
cooked beef or buffalo. You may want to add a bit of sugar to cut the
bitter taste. We never used to use sugar, of course, but when it came
along it was used by many.

❧ Buffaloberry Jelly

3 pounds of cleaned buffaloberries
1 cup water
3 cups sugar
1 package pectin

Cook the buffaloberries in the water. Add the sugar and cook 20 minutes more. Cool. Squeeze the fruit and liquid through a cloth. Put the
juice back on the stove on medium heat for another 20 minutes along
with the pectin. Follow the instructions on the pectin box. Fill three or
four sterilized pint jars. Cover with lids and rings, sealing and steril-
izing while hot.

❧ Buffaloberry Cream Cheese Spread

*This spread is not a traditional recipe at all. I just came up with it while working on
this book, but the results are really tasty. I think buffaloberry spread is really good
wrapped in a crunchy leaf of romaine lettuce. My editor, Lisa, thinks that it tastes
better with fresh coal cakes (little flatbreads) for breakfast. She would like to try it on
bagels some morning. Bill suggests that we should strain the seeds out, but Lisa and
I think they make a nice contrast to the smooth cream cheese.*

1 pint buffaloberries
2 tablespoons sugar
Water
8 ounces (or more) cream cheese

Place the berries and sugar in a saucepan and add water to just cover
the berries. Cook over medium heat until the berries are soft. Let the
mixture cool. Stir in the cream cheese until everything is well mixed
and smooth. If the spread is too runny, add more cream cheese.

⁛ Buffaloberry Ice Cream and Snow Cones

Sometimes when I was growing up, we would crush buffaloberries, mix canned milk with them, and put the container in the freezer. Before it was completely frozen we'd take it out and eat it. We'd call it ice cream, bullberry ice cream. Sometimes we made this ice cream with the buffaloberries and milk, but we would add snow and a little sugar too.

You can also mix just snow and sweetened berries for snow cones. Place the frosty mixture in cups and scoop it out with spoons.

Apples

Of course apples don't grow wild in Crow country, but they were already a favorite fruit by the time I was growing up. Bill has four apple trees that bear fruit. We have to watch out that bears and deer don't waste them. Back in the 1940s, baking an apple pie for your husband seemed to be a great way to show him you cared. Actually, it probably still is a pretty good way.

Apple Hollow Pie

When I was first married, living with Bill up at Fort Belknap, Montana, I really wanted to impress him, and I thought I was a pretty good cook. We had some dried apple rings that I had never seen before. I had plenty of experience with dried wild foods, so instead of telling Lena, Bill's aunt, that I didn't know what to do with them, I just pretended I knew and put them in a pie.

I made a real nice-looking pie and baked it until the top crust was all puffed up and a beautiful golden brown. I proudly placed it on the table, and as soon as Bill came in from a hard day's work, he smelled it, and I told him that we had apple pie for dessert. After the rest of the meal, he told me that he was ready for some pie. I cut him a slice and it was empty! All those dried apples were mushed together in a thin layer on the bottom.

Bill asked, "What is this, apple hollow pie?"

I cried.

His family laughed a lot about that pie, but I didn't think it was funny at the time.

Fortunately, Bill ate it anyway. "It's crusty, but it's nice," he said.

Soon Lena taught me how to use dried apples to make a good, full pie, but I have never forgotten that hollow one.

Beverages, Sweeteners, Thickeners, and Seasonings

Reading about drinks, sweeteners, thickeners, and flavorings, you'll see how Crow cuisine has changed over time.

Beverages

Water has always been the main drink of the Crow people. Elders tell us that rivers are like the veins of the world. They teach us to respect the waterways and to be thankful to the Creator every time we take a drink.

Clear, cool water from these creeks is good for a body. Nowadays, of course, Crow people drink pop, juice, milk, coffee, tea, and everything else just like everyone else, but I still think that plain, cool water is the best beverage for us.

Setting the Stage for Telling Tales

Plain water may be best for your health, but if you want a Crow person to tell you a story, I think you need to have hot drinks.

Awhile back, my grandson called and told me, "If you put on a really big pot of coffee, and get out some peaches and crackers, then I will come over and tell you some stories." The peaches and the crackers must be traditional; I know they are part of the Tobacco Ceremony. I'm not sure what they used in the old days before we had peaches—probably wild plums.

If you want me to tell stories, give me a cup of Earl Grey tea. It really calms me. If you want to hear *real* stories, don't let anyone interrupt or let the phone ring.

Pretty Shield never wasted any time. If she and other women were going to tell stories or sit around and talk, they'd all bring a craft to work on, and they'd have a cup of coffee or tea. They'd work on their crafts as they listened. So, for women, instead of sitting with a pipe and something to drink, telling stories, they'd have their craft work and something to drink, telling stories.

If Pretty Shield was rolling sinew into thread or pounding meat or berries, she would tell us stories or instructions as she worked. We were expected to learn what she was doing as well as what she was saying, and they would usually be two completely different things. We really had to pay attention to learn all she wanted to teach us.

Tea Time

Four "traditional" teas were drunk by the Crow people: mint, monarda, coyote, and catnip.

Mint tea was by far the most common. In fact, one of the Crow words for "mint" is the same as the word for "tea." We'd find mint (*Mentha arvensis*) in the Little Big Horn Valley. We'd pick a lot while we were there, use it fresh, and dry a little if there was extra. Picking mint was never something that we made a big project out of, and we never tried to dry a whole year's supply. We just picked it and used it up while we had it, and it was a nice change for a while. We weren't fussy about how we drank it either. If the tea was warm, we drank it warm with our bread. If it was leftover and cold, we drank it that way. We liked it either way. Most things were that way; leftovers were no problem with us.

In the mountains and along creeks you can find *aw wa xom bilish bi baba*, mountain mint (*Monarda fistulosa*), which is also called bee balm. It tastes like the bergamot that they use to flavor Earl Grey tea, which to me is a calming flavor.

I also heard about coyote mint tea (*chate ishbeleeshbita*) when I was growing up. It's made from a small, dark green plant with tiny leaves. I learned recently that this is pennyroyal (*Hedeoma hispida*). It's a plant with a lot of fresh minty flavor, and it really perks you up, but you should drink it only in moderation.

Sometimes women would get together and try different teas. Catnip was one of them. Some like it, some don't, and some can't stand the

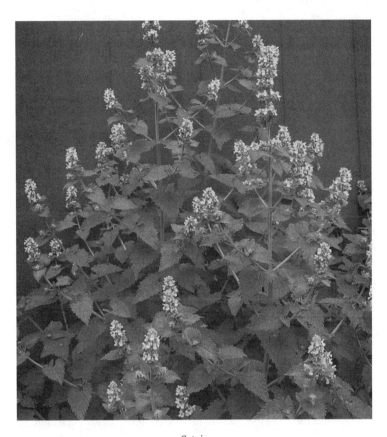

Catnip

smell if it's brewed too strong. I think it's calming, but I think of it more as medicine than as a nice drink to sit and sip.

Those teas are all from the mint family, and they all have square stems.

On occasion we'd drink other things that we called "teas" (*be lax a*) in Crow, but they were really fruit juices. We would get the juice out of chokecherries or any other berries and drink it, and we would call it tea. We would make the juice by cooking the berries and simply cooling off the juice. Nowadays if we don't make the juice for syrup, we just put it in the refrigerator.

Tea was probably more important in the old days, but by the time I was growing up, it seemed that all Crow people, even the children, were coffee drinkers.

ᶴ᷎ Wild Mint Tea

    1 quart water
    1 cup mint leaves and blossoms
    Honey or sugar (optional)

Boil the water and add the mint leaves and blossoms. Let set for 20 minutes. Add honey or sugar to taste, if desired. Serve.

ᶴ᷎ Wild Mint Blossoms and Black Tea

Mint makes a great tea all on its own (see the previous recipe), but it also blends well with black tea.

    1 quart water
    10 to 15 mint flowerheads
    3 or 4 tea bags of your favorite variety
    1/2 cup honey or sugar

Heat the water to a simmer and add the flowerheads. Simmer for 10 minutes. Remove from the heat. Add the tea bags and the honey or sugar. Let set until cool. Remove the tea bags and refrigerate the tea. When ready to serve, garnish each glass with a thin slice of lemon.

ᶴ᷎ Catnip Iced Tea

To make a refreshing summer drink from catnip, I add concentrated lemon juice and lots of ice.

    1 gallon water
    1 cup fresh catnip leaves (or 8 catnip tea bags)
    1 cup fresh or concentrated lemon juice (optional)
    3/4 cup sugar or honey (optional)

Boil the water and brew a strong tea with the catnip leaves or tea bags. Pour into a pitcher (mine holds 2 1/2 gallons) and add the lemon juice and sweetener, if desired. Fill the pitcher with water and ice and serve.

ᔟ Bitterberry Lemonade

From my friend Bonnie Heidel I learned that the orange-red berries of the bitterbush make a pretty orange lemonade-like drink. The berries from this foothills shrub (commonly called skunkbush, or aromatic sumac, Rhus aromatica) have a surprisingly citrus taste. Usually I use a tea made from bitterberries as a cosmetic or to ease the itching of poison ivy, but if you add enough sugar, it is pleasant to drink.

Cook a handful of bitterbush berries in 2 cups of water until the liquid turns a light orange. Strain and cool. Sweeten to taste and pour over ice.

Pretty Shield's Coffee

Pretty Shield, she was a coffee drinker. She would make a whole big pot of coffee, and I mean it was a big enamel coffee pot. It must have held three quarts. She'd get the water boiling and then throw a big handful of coffee in there. She didn't use a measure, just took a handful and threw it in. She didn't have a strainer either. Just water and coffee grounds all together. When she'd get done boiling it, my, she'd enjoy her coffee. She did sweeten it a bit. She didn't put cream or anything else in it, but she did sweeten it a little bit.

If there was any coffee left, she would keep it cold. And then the next morning, she'd heat the same pot and drink it again. She never hollered for fresh coffee. She saved it.

Her storytelling buddy was Frank Linderman, who talked to her and wrote the book *Pretty-Shield: Medicine Woman of the Crows.* My older sister, Cerise, told me that Pretty Shield would pour coffee for Frank Linderman, and he would say, "I love your coffee, Pretty Shield. It's the strongest coffee around, and that's the way I like it." And he would drink coffee with her, those old timers.

Later, black tea came along. It was loose tea, not ground leaves done up in these little packages. Pretty Shield would do the same thing with that tea that she did with her coffee. She would boil a pot of water, and when it was hot, she'd pick up a few of those tea leaves and put them in the water. It came out all right. It tasted like regular black tea, but we were used to drinking tea that was green from all the mint.

Sometimes when I was young, the food situation was really desperate at our place. My brothers and sisters tell me that Pretty Shield used to feed me coffee from a spoon after my mother died. There was not always enough milk. I drank canned milk when there was. I remember the milk—it was Carnation, in a red and white can. Amongst themselves my brothers and sisters would collect nickels and dimes and other things to get me milk. They'd mix the canned milk half and half with water, and they'd feed it to me. That was my milk. I never knew a bottle. I was fed mostly with spoons but also, sometimes, with some udder of a cow or buffalo. They'd take the udder and cut a long piece from it. They would dunk it in milk, and I'd suck it and dunk it in the milk and suck it until I was old enough to go to spoons. I wasn't too much on the sucking part because I was already a year and a half old then, but they fed me that way because of a lack of implements, I guess. Then they'd spoon stuff to me, and coffee was one of the things that Pretty Shield would give me when I'd cry and they didn't have milk. That's when they would all take the nickel and dime collection to buy me a can of milk.

Sweeteners

Honey

Sugar wasn't always plentiful when I was growing up. You couldn't just go down to the store and get more. So my father, who was pretty independent, would collect his own honey. He'd go down to the big cottonwood trees along the river, the Little Big Horn River, there near where he lived at Benteen.

He didn't seem to do anything special. He just tapped the trees and filled up one of his great big round tubs two-thirds full of honey and wax. The wax would float on top of the honey. He'd let us take a piece of wax, and we'd chew it like chewing gum. It was sweet and tasted of the honey. Even after the sweet taste was gone, and the wax was almost pure white, we'd chew it like gum, just to be chewing.

Dad would then use the honey for everything. If he was baking a cake—and he was a good baker—he'd use honey wherever a recipe called for sugar.

I don't remember Dad getting in much trouble with the bees while he was collecting the honey. I really don't remember there being any great quantity of bees around. In fact, sometimes he tried to get the bees to sting him. He had arthritic wrists, and he thought that a bee sting would help ease the pain and loosen the joint. So he tried to provoke the bees to attack him. I don't know if it worked, and I didn't stay around to watch my daddy get stung by bees. I didn't want to see that.

Other sweeteners that we could get around here were even harder to come by, before sugar was common. People mostly used fruit, which isn't always all that sweet. Sometimes the ground tomatoes, bitgup awda (Physalis pumila), were used to thicken and sweeten up a stew or sauce. If you suck the end of a blossom of ba a ba li chi gua gat tay, you can get a drop of sweet nectar. No quantity enough to cook with can be collected, but for kids walking by and picking the flower, it was always a sweet treat. (The English name for this flower is Indian paintbrush, but of course we did not call them that. The genus name for the several species is Castilleja.) Northwest of here, the Rocky Boys Indians collected sweet sap from the box elder (bishpe) in the early spring and used it as a sweetener. Box elder (Acer negundo) is in the maple family, so the taste of the sap is a lot like maple syrup, only a bit clearer.

Thickeners

Making puddings and sauces requires something to thicken the fruit. The easiest thing these days is just to add cornstarch, tapioca, or flour. Before they were readily available we had the options of ehe (wild turnip), ground tomatoes, and sego lilies.

Sego lilies (minmo baba leegisha, the Calochortus species) have edible roots that can be dried and made into flour. The small white three-sided lily flowers with their little yellow centers are gorgeous out here on the hillsides, but I'm not in the habit of using them for food. It seems that every time I dig one, all that comes up is this little tiny root not worth fussing about. My sister Cerise uses them, however, and she makes flour from the root and uses it as a thickener.

Seasonings

Long ago the food around here was very simple. It was mostly just the meat, berries, and vegetables. Some used sage or mint for seasoning, others chose prairie onions or cedar berries. It was never too much.

When I was growing up, Pretty Shield certainly used salt and really liked sugar, but she never caught on to these spices and herbs in little jars. My sisters and sometimes even my father would try new seasonings, but Pretty Shield liked to use just her few wild plants and not much else.

I have a whole cupboard full of jars now, and I've always been open to trying new spices. Still, most of the time I stick to my favorites: pepper, some herb blends, and bay leaves for stews (even though traditionally it was mint that went into dry-meat stews). I've also found some wonderful wild seasoning plants around here. Three weedy plants in the mustard family have a peppery taste, and we call them all *aw wa xosh she bita*, "peppers." Little peppergrass (*Lepidium* species) has round, ball-shaped seedheads. Shepherd's purse (*Capsella bursa-pastoris*) is just a bit taller with seedheads that look like hearts. My favorite of the three is penny cress (*Thlaspi arvense*), which is taller yet and has seedheads more like flattened hearts. Its seeds are peppery, like the others, but they have a bit of a garlic taste to them as well. Try all of these in recipes instead of black pepper. Add a taste of the wild as well as a taste of heritage.

2

Meats

When we walk in step with nature, she provides the roots and fruits that we need for our nutrients, but without hunting buffalo and other game, the Crow people would never have survived life on the plains. Here I have collected stories and recipes about the essential buffalo and other meats I've tried.

Buffalo: Bíshǎ Bison

The buffalo (or as my scientist friends remind me, the American bison) has always been important to the Crow people. Pretty Shield told fabulous tales of following the buffalo herds and of raising a buffalo calf. (Read the stories for yourself in her book *Pretty-Shield: Medicine Woman of the Crows*.) Her storytelling buddy, Frank Linderman, once asked her why she had no stories about the time after the tribe followed the buffalo. Pretty Shield told him that there was nothing to say. Nothing was worth talking about once they had moved to the reservation and stopped following the buffalo. When she was living on the reservation, she told him, "Everything was so beautiful to me; I loved our moves, and we went anywhere we chose. Now there is ugly wire all around us; we are like trapped animals." Buffalo represent freedom to the Crow people. They are that important to the Crow people.

Even now when most Crow people eat more beef than buffalo (beef is a lot easier to come by, and we seem to have developed a taste for it), buffalo is still the best meat for special occasions. If I were to hold a feast for a wedding or prepare some other special dinner, I would serve ribs, baked buffalo ribs. I'd also have boiled red potatoes with parsley, corn on the cob, and a big green salad. Of course there would be some kind of bread, but it wouldn't have to be fry bread. I prefer a good black bread. We'd have coffee and tea and pies made with juneberries and huckleberries afterward, but the buffalo would be the main dish.

I like the taste, so if I can get it, I will have buffalo anytime. I do not need to wait for a special feast.

Let me remind you of something. Buffalo are very important to the Crow people; however, the Crow people have never worshiped the buffalo. Respect and worship are different things. I thank the buffalo for feeding us, and I respect their strength and power, but I worship God, the Creator. Buffalo are not and have never been gods.

I never followed the buffalo on the open range the way that Pretty Shield did, so I do not have as many stories about them as she did. But I do remember her roasting buffalo liver on coals, preparing the many-folds cleaned fresh out of the animal, and boiling the hooves with corn.

Liver

Pretty Shield used to throw a liver, just as it was—fresh from the animal—into hot coals. The outer layer would sear right away, and then the inside would cook slowly. An hour (if she used half the liver of a buffalo or cow) or an hour and a half later, she'd take it out, brush off the ashes, slice it, and call us to come and eat.

The top part was so crusty that we'd just hold it with our fingers and eat out the inside. It was warm and smooth. It tasted like liver pâté, and it was really good with a biscuit and some tea.

Many-folds: Ishbaubay

"Many-folds" is an edible part of a cow or buffalo that the Crows use. It is an organ that is involved with digestion, but it is not the tripe, and it has many folds. I would say it is like a big football whose surface has many folds instead of just being smooth. The organ is attached on its ends and in between the attachment points, there are many folds. In each fold you can see the grass that the animal has eaten. It's still there, and the grass still looks like grass.

Of course, you have to wash out the grass. Throw the whole thing in the creek and just wash it. Wash every fold. When I was growing up, some women washed the folds so clean that they became white. Others washed the many folds very well, but they left the thin skin on it so the folds remained a sort of grayish green.

It cooks well. It cooks very tender. And when it is tender, it is very tasty.

When the men were in the process of butchering, and Grandma was cleaning up that many-folds, we kids would go over there, and we didn't want to wait. "We're hungry," we would whine. So Pretty Shield would clean the many-folds first. It took a while for her to clean it, so we would have to help. Then she would rub it so the grayish-green skin would come off. That would leave the many-folds white. Well, whitish-pink— a light, light pink.

Pretty Shield would tear off one fold. The piece would be about a half inch wide and seven inches long. She would tie a knot at one end. Then she would tie another knot just below that knot and another and another until the whole thing was a row of knots with a little space between each one.

Then she would give us the knotted fold, and we would have to bite off the first knot. We would chew and chew and chew. We'd chew until we had the knot all chewed up, and only then did we swallow it. The reason she knotted the fold is that some people would eat and swallow the string whole, real fast, but it wouldn't digest when eaten that way. It would come out unchanged in the bowel, and they were afraid to pull it out. Anyone who ate a whole fold would have to sit there until it worked itself out. Of course we didn't want that, so we would chew just as Pretty Shield told us to.

So, after she knotted the many-folds, we would have to chew the knots so they would be well chewed in our mouths before we swallowed. That way the fold would digest well, and we would get the value of the food, rather than just letting it slide through.

In general, Pretty Shield thought that chewing food was important. She always said, "Chew your food well so that your stomach will not ache, and you won't have cramps. And drink lots of water." We didn't drink much water right with the food, but we did after we ate.

Boiled Hooves

Pretty Shield would take the hooves of buffalo, scrape them, and tap out the debris. Then she would wash them and put them in boiling water. When it looked like the hooves were without dirt and debris, she would change the water. She would change the water, bring it to a boil again, and put the hooves back in. Then she would boil and boil them for most of the afternoon. After that she would take them out, and she would skin them. She would skin the hide off the hooves. I never saw Pretty Shield do anything with the hide from the hooves. Some people make baskets with it, but I don't know how. Pretty Shield would take that skin off, and then she would wash the hooves again. She would change the water, boil some fresh water. Then she would put the skinned hooves back in and let them boil the rest of the afternoon. When she took them out after that boiling, the collagen on the hooves slipped right out, and that's when they were good to go ahead and eat.

A long time ago, that actual hard part that slips right off, the Crows would use for water containers or rattles. I never saw Pretty Shield do anything with them though. But the rest of the hooves, boy, did they taste good. She would cook them until they gelled. We loved to eat them. She would put corn in with them, corn taken off the cobs. She would put corn and squash in there. And when that was done, it was perfect eating.

Pretty Shield always told us that the hooves of the animal would give us good healthy hair and would replenish and lubricate our joints.

Marrow from the bones we believed did the same thing. It would go to the joints and make them work well, grease them up. Marrow would also grease the lining of the stomach to keep it healthy.

I have a great alternative to potato chips for the times you're sitting in front of the television. They're crunchy, like chips, and go down easy, but they're much lower in fat and higher in protein. They're dried buffalo lungs. Good snacking and good for you.

You don't need to boil hooves all day, tie knots in many-folds, or even dry buffalo lungs (although I really do recommend them) to try buffalo. It can be cooked in any number of different ways. Here are a few of my favorites to try.

🐄 Wild Buffalo Boiled with Vegetables

2 pounds buffalo meat, cut into 2-inch chunks
2 gallons water
2 bay leaves
1 small onion, chopped
2 large or 3 small carrots, cut up
2 cups celery, cut into 1-inch lengths
6 medium potatoes, quartered
Salt and pepper to taste

In a stainless steel pot, boil the meat for one hour in the water with the bay leaves. Add the onion, carrots, celery, potatoes, salt, and pepper. Cook another half an hour.

Serves 8.

❧ Buffalo Tenderloin and Kidneys

My grandfather, Goes Ahead, told my brother not to eat kidneys, but in general Crow people eat and enjoy almost all of an animal.

2 pounds buffalo tenderloin
2 buffalo kidneys
1 onion, chopped
1 cup canned, sliced mushrooms
Salt and pepper
$^1/_4$ cup flour
1 quart water

Cut the tenderloin and kidneys into bite-sized pieces. Sear them in an oiled skillet until browned. Add the onion and mushrooms. Season with salt and pepper to taste. Sprinkle the flour over the mixture, stirring until blended. Add one quart of water. Simmer until tender, about 1 hour. Serve over mashed potatoes or rice.

Serves 8 to 10.

❧ Buffalo Ribs

8 buffalo short ribs
4 bay leaves
4 to 5 cloves garlic, sliced or chopped
1 medium onion chopped or 1 tablespoon dehydrated onion

Cut the buffalo ribs into short pieces. Place the ribs on a rack in a roasting pan and bake for 1 hour, uncovered. Remove the ribs and cover the bottom of the pan with a small amount of water. Add the bay leaves. Sprinkle the ribs with the garlic and onion. Cover and bake for another hour. Baste the ribs with the pan juice, placing the bay leaves between the ribs. Cover and cook another half hour. Baste the ribs well. Test the ribs and continue roasting them until they are tender. When done, serve with toasted bread.

Serves 8.

❧ Seasoned Ground Buffalo Patties

2 pounds ground buffalo meat
1 medium onion, chopped
1 egg
1 teaspoon salt
1/8 teaspoon pepper
1 can tomatoes (14.5 ounces)
1 teaspoon vinegar
1 1/2 cups water, divided
1/2 cup raisins, juneberries, or grapes
1 1/2 teaspoons curry powder
1 teaspoon cinnamon
1 1/2 teaspoons flour

Combine the meat, onion, egg, salt, pepper, tomatoes, and vinegar. Shape the mixture into small flattened meatballs. Brown in a hot skillet. Pour off the excess grease and remove the patties. Combine 1/2 cup of warm water with the raisins and set aside until the raisins are soft. Mix the curry powder, cinnamon, and flour in a skillet and then pour in 1 cup of water and mix. Add the buffalo patties and raisins and cook until thickened. Serve over mashed potatoes or biscuits.

Serves 8.

❧ Charcoal-Baked Liver

Wash a whole liver, with its skin still on, and dry it off. (You may instead use half a liver, if you wish.) Make a cottonwood or box-elder fire and let it burn down to about three inches of hot coals. Lay the liver on the coals and sweep more coals over the liver until it's completely covered. Leave for approximately half an hour and then check that the liver is still covered with hot coals. Check again after about 1 hour. Take the liver out of the coals and slice it to see if it is cooked. When it's done, sweep the ashes off the liver and place it on a cutting board. Allow it to set for 10 minutes to make slicing easy. Slice the liver and make sandwiches with it or serve it as an entrée. Wild carrots with a dash of wild pepper (see Wild Vegetables as well as Seasonings in chapter 1) make a nice accompaniment.

❧ Crushed Buffalo Bone Soup, Traditional Style

Lay out a clean tarp on the ground and place a large, flat rock in the middle. Pound marrow bones against the rock with a tomahawk-type (rock) mallet or maul. When the pounding is completed, remove the rock, gather up the tarp, and pour the bone pieces into a 4-quart (or larger) iron kettle. Pour water over the bones to cover them. Boil for 2 hours. Strain off the broth and add salt and pepper. You can also mix the broth with pounded jerky or crushed wild berries or both.

❧ Crushed Buffalo Bone Soup, Modern Style

Floating fat, also called membrane fat, is found between membrane layers on a buffalo. Using floating fat or kidney fat makes this recipe more authentic, but bacon fat can easily be substituted.

$^1/_2$ pound jerky, cut in strips

2 cups dried squash, broken into 1-inch pieces

1 cup wild turnip roots, chopped or sliced

2 cups dried corn or canned hominy

2 tablespoons honey or $^1/_4$ cup corn syrup

Piece of floating fat, kidney fat, or bacon fat, about 2 x 3 inches

2 quarts water

Salt and pepper

3 tablespoons flour, approximately (optional)

Place the jerky, squash, turnips, dried corn, honey, and floating fat in boiling water and cook until the jerky is tender, approximately 2 $^1/_2$ hours. Add more water, if necessary. Season with salt and pepper according to your taste. You can stir in the flour to thicken the soup, if you like, but I usually don't.

Serves about 4.

A TASTE OF HERITAGE FOODS

❧ Dried Lungs

Slice the lungs ¹/₄ inch thick as you would for jerky. If possible, leave the whole side of a lung together. Place over a horizontal pole to dry in the sun. Usually poles are erected clothesline style when they are used for dehydrating foodstuffs. Bring the lungs in during the night and rehang during the day until completely dry and crispy. The lungs are taffy colored when they are dry. Then place them on a rack over hot coals or bake in a 350-degree oven for approximately 10 minutes to make them nicer to eat. Wash the drying poles or racks after use. The dried lungs will keep as long as jerky will, for about a year or so.

❧ Jerky and Fatback

1 pound fatback (salt pork) or bacon, cut in chunks
2 quarts water
1 pound plain jerky
2 tablespoons dehydrated onion or 1 medium onion, chopped
1 can yellow hominy
3 pounds red or white potatoes (red potatoes are best)
Pepper, to taste

Trim the rind off the fatback and cut the meat into pieces. Bring the water to a boil in a nonaluminum three-quart saucepan. Add the salt pork and jerky. Boil for 1 ¹/₂ hours. Add the onion, hominy, and potatoes. Cook another 45 minutes. If desired, add pepper. This stew is good served with wheel bread.

Serves 6 to 8.

❧ Marrow Gut, Three Ways

Very soon after butchering, Grandma used to serve us the marrow gut, the curly intestine of a buffalo or cow. Here I offer three ways to cook and serve it.

First, cut the marrow gut into several separate lengths and wash thoroughly with several changes of water until the strips are clean and pale in color.

Method 1: Cut the marrow gut into 5-inch lengths, roll them in seasoned flour, and fry in hot grease until nicely browned. Lower the heat and continue slowly frying for approximately half an hour, or until tender. Serve with crackers or baking-powder bread.

Method 2: Cut the marrow gut into small pieces and boil with other cuts of buffalo or beef until tender.

Method 3: Take three lengths (about one foot long each) of the marrow gut and tie them together at one end with butcher's string. Braid the three sections together and tie the end with more string. Lower the braid into boiling water for about one hour, or until tender. Serve on a platter, letting everyone cut off their own portion.

❧ Buffalo Marrow

Extracting marrow from a cooked animal bone that is not split is very difficult, but it can be done. In the old days, Indians took a skewer or a peeled chokecherry twig and inserted it into the end of the bone and pulled the marrow out. It was either eaten directly off the utensil or with meat or bread. Some people immersed the marrow in boiling salted water for a few minutes and then put it on bread. Marrow looks like fat; it's soft, off-white in color, and can be spread like peanut butter.

❧ Buffalo Cooked in a Parfleche

I've never myself cooked with hot rocks and meat in a parfleche. A parfleche is the untanned hide of an animal without the hair—rawhide—and it can withstand heat and won't leak. Pretty Shield told me about this old way of cooking. Even if preparing meat is easier now, Pretty Shield told me that it was faster with hot rocks. When everything was readied beforehand, it took only seven minutes to actually cook the meat.

A TASTE OF HERITAGE FOODS

Meat was placed in a parfleche with already hot water and hot rocks. The parfleche was hung on a tripod over more hot rocks. The water would boil, and they'd take out the rocks with tongs, usually a forked choke-cherry stick. They'd replace the cooking rocks as soon as possible with more hot rocks in order to keep the water boiling and really hot.

All the Rest of the Buffalo Parts

Even if you think you don't care for any of the recipes that I have offered in this chapter, a buffalo could still come in handy. Here are some examples of things the Crow Indians and some other groups of Plains Indians did with the rest of the buffalo.

Hide

Buffalo hide was used for shelter as well as for clothes, ropes, boats, rugs, and blankets. The tanned hide was obviously the very important covering of the lodge. Smaller pieces of hide were used for lining the teepee. This lining extended from halfway up the teepee down to the floor, where the beds and parfleches (clothes boxes) were placed.

The thick hump hair of the buffalo was used for baby comfort and for feminine hygiene purposes. The hair and shavings of the hide were also used to stuff pillows and for playthings that required stuffing.

Fat

An elderly lady of the Assiniboine tribe taught me that during the dressing out of a buffalo, a container should be placed under a small opening at the front end of the hump. She explained that while she worked the hump, the fat from it, which is unsaturated, would fill the container. This fat did not solidify and was good to eat mixed with crushed berries and jerky.

Jerky Meat

Jerky was one of the main foods used by the Indian tribes of the Plains. Jerky is made by thinly slicing pieces of meat and drying them in the sun. In the buffalo days, all women set up racks for drying meat near their tipis.

They prepared the dried meat for eating in several ways. After it was cooked over flames, it was eaten in chunks or pounded. Usually the pounded jerky was mixed with fat before it was consumed. If the jerky was to be kept for long periods of time, tallow from around the kidney was used as a preservative. Kidney fat does not spoil as other fats do. To prepare pounded meat, mix 5 cups of meat to 1 cup of tallow. Tallow used for pemmican was hidden in cool, dark places, where it would keep for months. Jerky was also boiled with canned corn, canned hominy, or wild rice. These dishes were usually served with wheel bread and tea.

Heart, Kidneys, and Liver

After a buffalo was killed, the heart, kidneys, and liver were eaten first, while they were fresh and warm. The heart (of a buffalo or any other animal) was never eaten raw, but the kidneys and liver were sometimes relished that way. Most often, however, all these internal organs were prepared by roasting them over hot coals.

Entrails

All the entrails of a buffalo were eaten, except for the last foot of colon gut, and it was thrown away along with the private parts.

Bladder

The bladder was used to carry water, or it was painted, filled with deer hair, and used as a ball by children.

Rib Bones

Rib bones would be bleached in the sun and used to make tools, or they might be cut into pieces and used in various games and crafts.

Leg-bone Marrow

Marrow extracted from leg bones was considered a delicacy to be mixed with berries or eaten with cooked meat or jerky for nourishment. Bones were crushed, boiled, and strained. When the resulting liquid cooled, the marrow fat hardened at the top of the container. Moderns call this marrow fat "Indian butter."

Hooves

In addition to boiling hooves and serving them with corn, Crow Indians also prepared buffalo hooves in a manner similar to pickled pigs' feet, except no vinegar solution was used. Then they would be cooked in a stew with vegetables.

I once fleetingly saw hooves used another way in a display. The children of Upper Peninsula Indians of the Great Lakes area at one time wore colorful, decorated hooves for shoes. The museum is in Sault Ste. Marie, Michigan.

Shoulder Blades

The fan-shaped bones that form the shoulder blades of a buffalo were used as containers for preparing food and for mixing the plant materials that would be burned in a pipe. They were also used as plates or scoops.

Milk Bag

When a cow buffalo was slaughtered, the Crows took the milk bag from the animal and cut it in strips. It's very, very tough. They cut it and let babies suck on the strips.

Tendons

The sinew from a tendon near the backbone of the animal was cut off and while still soft was used for teething babies along with the milk-bag strips. Of course, dried sinew provided thread for sewing many things.

Tongue

Tongue was a delicacy that was used in ceremonies like the Sun Dance. Grandmother Pretty Shield always mentioned that a proper Sun Dance had ninety slices of buffalo tongue strung up and hung from one end of the Sun Dance lodge to the other.

Head

Sun dancers mounted a buffalo head, except for the tongue and brains, on the center pole of the Sun Dance lodge.

Horns

Dippers and scrapers were made from buffalo horns, and men used them for crafts as well.

Brain

The most important use for buffalo brains was to soften hides during tanning.

Other Meats

Choice Meats

Different meats are good for different things. Buffalo is generally the best meat all around. It makes the best boiled meat, I would say, and it makes the best dried meat and stew too. Buffalo ribs roasted with bay leaves, coarse pepper, and salt are delicious. I consider buffalo and beef both great for steaks. The only thing that keeps me from turning completely to beef are the chemicals. As far as taste goes, I prefer beef steaks. For roasts, I would say that elk is my favorite. For frying, I would say deer tenderloin steaks. So what's best depends on how you use the meat.

Growing up, we didn't have many choices. Occasionally while we were growing up, we'd get some buffalo, and Pretty Shield would make jerky or pemmican. But there wasn't always buffalo available. Pretty Shield would get Goes Ahead's pension check the first of every month, and she would go to the store and buy good beef. So during the first part of the month, we'd always have beef from the store. Then after that, we relied on deer more than anything. We'd get by on deer and elk and rabbits, lots of rabbits, and the occasional prairie chicken.

Beef: Bíshá e geelay

Pretty Shield had a hard time adjusting to beef because she always ate buffalo as a child. She hated beef at first—couldn't stand the smell of it. But she got used to it when she had to, and she learned to cook it really well.

My father would kill a longhorn every fall for Pretty Shield. A lot of people would come around for the entrails and other delicacies. You

A TASTE OF HERITAGE FOODS

can't keep those long. They need to be eaten fresh. He'd slaughter the animal right alongside the river, where the entrails could be washed right and quickly.

I never knew what happened to the longhorn hide. My grandmother never fooled with the hide of a cow. But some people would use them.

One time they killed a cow in my uncle's yard. There was an old man whose name was Bad Heart. Once when they had a kill right there in my uncle's yard, Bad Heart went over with a cup. When they cut the jugular vein, he filled his cup and drank the blood just like that. He was the first and only person I have seen drink the blood, but my dad told me that they did that in the old days.

After a cow was butchered, people started eating on it right away. The brain was fried in oil. The liver was thrown into hot coals to make a "liver pâté," the way buffalo liver was traditionally cooked. The ribs were boiled in water, and the resulting broth was relished. When they sliced the big pieces of meat for making jerky, a few slices were thrown on a hot grill and cooked like barbecue. The rest of the meat was immediately hung to dry. The flank was hung in a semidry place to be fried later.

You can substitute beef for buffalo in the recipes on the previous pages, although the results will not taste quite the same.

Deer: Ooh xaa

Growing up we ate a lot of deer—mule deer and white-tailed deer—because they could be hunted from the wild. Deer meat is always good fried or boiled, and deer ribs were boiled and saved for good eating later, served either warm or cold.

Deer hides make very soft moccasins and dresses. I once tanned about six deer hides, and the skin was all nice and soft. I did this when I was up north with my husband Bill's people. Bill's grandma showed me how to do it. Tanning hides was not that hard to do, but patience was required. I soaked the deer hides in Fels Naptha soap and water. This step took a long time. I checked the hides daily, and finally the hair would almost drop off with just a gentle pull. After I pulled all the hair off, we wrung out the hides to get rid of the water and then put them through a handmade scraper that was attached to a tree. The scraper was made out of a toothed rod that was shaped like a half moon, and it was fastened on each end to the tree. Grandma Buck would put the buckskin in between the tree and the blade, threading it in and around, and then she showed me how to pull the skin back and forth, back and forth. It was long, tedious work.

Pretty Shield taught me another way to tan. She taught all of us girls how to do it, but then you had to have more than one person to do it her way. Since there were always more than a couple of girls around, she'd have us work together, stretching the hide in a circular motion. Pull and move, pull and move, pull and move, until the skin dried that way, nice and strong.

Tanning hides the Fort Belknap way, I made six deerskins, and I gave them all to my sister Cerise. I was very proud of them, and she was very proud of them when I gave them to her. She put them to her face to feel how soft they were. I gave them to her for her moccasins. I don't know if I could ever tan deer hides again, just because it was such tedious work.

ꜟ Deer Steaks

This recipe is simple, but it really tastes good.

Slice deer meat about half an inch thick. Coat the meat with flour, salt, and pepper. Heat a griddle or skillet to medium-high with just enough oil to brown the meat. Place the meat in the pan and cook until desired doneness. I like my deer meat well done, which takes about 7 minutes on each side. Serve the steaks with mustard or steak sauce. If there is some plum ketchup or buffaloberries around, the steaks would taste so much better.

A TASTE OF HERITAGE FOODS

Elk: Egeligosha

Elk meat is very good dried, and it makes excellent roasts. A lot of elk live in both Absalooka (Crow) country and Assiniboine country, where my husband's people are. The hunters travel to the mountains to hunt and usually take a couple days.

⏁ Elk Roast

Salt and pepper an elk roast. Place it in a heavy pan or roasting oven, cover it, and roast in a 350-degree oven for 45 minutes per pound. Slices of elk roast served between two warm coal cakes make delicious sandwiches (see the coal cake version of the wheel bread recipe in chapter 3).

Antelope: Aapkaxxe

Antelope meat can be very wild tasting. It can taste too much like the sage that the pronghorn antelope live among. Crow hunters were taught not to kill an antelope if it runs away but rather only to shoot those that they could sneak up on. My husband Bill says that if you don't run antelope, they make good eating. Also, as soon as you slaughter an antelope, remove the glands at the back of the legs. This will improve the flavor of the meat.

I like the meat cooked with garlic and salt and pepper, and as I often do with other game meats, I marinate it in beef bouillon before cooking it to take the antelope taste down a bit. Antelope makes good dried meat too.

⏁ Bill's Mother's Antelope Roast

My husband's mother, Hazel, lived with us for a while, and she cooked antelope meat. She roasted a well-seasoned antelope roast in the oven. When it was nearly done she took the cover off and let it brown. She also basted it while it was cooking, and I noticed slices of onions all over the roast while she was doing this. She used garlic and tomato sauce to make a good gravy. It was delicious.

If I were fixing this antelope roast, I would set the oven at 350 degrees and allow about 45 minutes of cooking time for every pound of meat.

At different times during my life, I have tried all sorts of meats. These days we pretty much stick to what we can get at the grocery store, but when you had to hunt food for your family, you would eat whatever you could catch.

Moose: Apashbia

We never had many moose down around Crow. Up north in Fort Belknap a moose would come around once in a while. But usually we'd get moose and moose hides from Canada. Visiting tribes would bring them down even as far as Crow to sell.

Some people like moose meat better than elk meat. I would say it's a little sweeter in flavor than elk or deer.

Whenever we get a hide to tan from a moose, we like it because their hides seem to have "threads" that run in just one direction and are easier to work. Deer hides are harder to punch needles through because the threads in their hides are crisscrossed. Deer hide is very, very soft. Elk hide is wonderfully soft too. But tanning work is fastest with moose hide.

Moose hides are often used for moccasins, and I am in the process of making a robe with one.

❧ Old-time Moose Roast

Roasting moose meat in the ground in the old way gives it the best flavor.

Dig a hole three feet deep and ten inches across. Place hot rocks in the bottom. Place whole skunk cabbage leaves (or a little sage or juniper, if you don't have skunk cabbage) on the hot rocks along with a little water. Put in more hot rocks, more leaves, and then chunks of moose meat, more leaves, and more meat. Top the meat with a layer of rocks. Then close up the hole with a piece of rawhide. Cover it with soil and weigh it down with rocks. Leave the meat to cook all day. Take the meat out and enjoy.

Rabbit: Eesush bit sheela

Rabbit. We ate rabbit a lot. It wasn't anything special. We'd just boil the rabbit and put vegetables in with it. Sometimes we fried rabbits very slowly or baked them, and they were very good. I think they're best cut in sections, floured, and fried.

When I was young we had only wild rabbits. Later on, Bill and I went to visit his real mother in Oregon. Her husband at that time raised rabbits. We would have them fixed all kinds of ways over there. And I dare say that, to me, tame rabbits taste much better than the wild rabbits. I don't know why, but I like them much better. They have such nice white meat.

There's an old Crow warning that says if you eat rabbit when you're pregnant, your baby will be born with a cleft palate. I don't know if it's true, but Pretty Shield really believed it.

Beaver: Bee laubã

Beaver had many uses for the Crow people. Besides making necklaces out of the beaver musk for her grandsons, Pretty Shield probably rubbed beaver oil into our hair.

Crow people also used beaver pelts, and we'd eat only the beaver tail. Beaver tail is good. It consists of a real milky fat and is very different.

Over in Michigan the Chippewas cook and eat the whole beaver body but not the tail. Isn't that funny? When Bill and I were there, I ate some of the flesh, and it was surprisingly very good. It was almost like beef but a little sweeter. They seasoned it well. I think it was spiced with rosemary.

❧ Beaver Tail

Here's a recipe in case you ever come across a beaver tail you want to eat. I don't know of any seasoning, not even mint leaves, used with beaver tail, but I think that cedar or rosemary would give good flavor to it.

1 beaver tail
Seasonings

Place the beaver tail in a pot with water to cover it entirely. Cook over high heat for about 2 hours, checking to see that the water level stays above the tail. Then leave the tail cooking over medium heat for an afternoon. Take the tail out of the water and skin it. Slice and serve with meat, a sauce of berries, and wheel bread. Beaver tail is good tasting, chewy, and rich.

Bear: Dax bitcha

Black bears and brown bears live in Crow country. Black bear is not a traditional Crow food, but we have eaten it. I have fixed it myself—I roasted it. Bear has a sweet taste.

Bighorn Sheep and Mountain Goats: Aoxaxbutaga and Esabuataga

My brother's mother-in-law boiled bighorn sheep just plain. Sheep and mountain goats are the kinds of animals you eat only when you are desperate. When you are hungry, you need no spices.

❧ Mint Sauce for Modern Lamb Chops

While I did not eat them growing up, and I still don't eat them often, I have grown to appreciate a good lamb chop. I developed this sauce to show off the flavors of the local plants and bring out the sweetness in the lamb.

¹/₂ cup bone marrow or margarine
¹/₂ cup Indian lettuce, chopped
1 cup watercress, chopped
1 cup wild mint, chopped
2 cups water
1 teaspoon vinegar
1 cup honey
¹/₂ cup wild grape juice

Boil the bone marrow, Indian lettuce, watercress, mint, and water until the leaves are tender. Mix in the vinegar, honey, and wild grape juice. Simmer for another 5 minutes. Pour over lamb chops and bake until the chops are done, about 1 hour.

Fish, Fowl, and Eggs

Fish, fowl, and eggs have never been all that important to the Crow people, but they make up more of our diets these days.

Fish: Bwah

While the Big Horn and Little Big Horn Rivers that run through Crow country are full of trout, the Crow did not eat them very often. My brother George, however, used to love to fish. He'd go out and catch fish using just old safety pins for hooks. He caught a lot, but he never ate them in our house. Pretty Shield couldn't stand to be around fish. She had been told not to eat fish, and she didn't. Who told her that, I don't know. I don't know why anyone would have told her that. Maybe she was allergic to fish.

I learned to eat fish after I married Bill. We have it more often now because it is so healthy, and fish tastes so good with many of the wild seasonings from around here.

ఊ Trout, Local Style

I created this recipe to show off foods from here in the Big Horn Valley, even though they weren't traditionally served together.

Pick some wild lettuce (the Montia species, also called Indian lettuce or miner's lettuce). Pick some watercress. Rinse and thoroughly clean the two vegetables. Wrap a filet of trout in the leaves and then wrap fish and leaves together in aluminum foil. Place the packet on the coals of an open fire. Cook until the fish is opaque and flaky. Slice open some already baked push bread and eat the fish and greens in the bread.

ఊ Stuffed Trout

At a presentation I gave in Wyoming, this stuffed trout was a big hit among the boys. The girls tried it politely, but the boys, they just loved it and even asked to keep the leftovers. That worked out great because it saved me packing it up and driving it home.

3 pounds rainbow trout
2 cups wild rice
1 quart water
1 cup carrots, diced
2 cups celery, diced
1 onion, diced
4 cups dried bread crumbs
Salt to taste
1 tablespoon parsley
$1/2$ cup soybean oil
2 cups soy milk
1 tablespoon sage
2 eggs

Clean the trout and place them in salt water in the refrigerator either overnight or at least 4 hours before stuffing.

Put the wild rice in the quart of boiling water and cook for 1 $1/2$ hours. When done, set aside to cool. Add the diced carrots, celery, and onion.

In a large bowl, mix together the bread crumbs, salt, parsley, soybean oil, and soy milk. Stir until well blended. Add the sage and stir

A TASTE OF HERITAGE FOODS

again. Combine the wild rice mixture with the bread crumb mixture. Scramble the eggs. Add the scrambled eggs to the stuffing.

Rinse the saltiness from the fish in fresh running water. Use the stuffing mixture to stuff the trout. Place them in an oblong baking dish and bake at 350 degrees for 45 minutes.

This recipe makes plenty of stuffing, so stuff the fish pretty full. The way I served it gave 12 people a small taste. It would probably feed 6 as an entrée.

Gourmet Smorgasbord Fish

For a while in the early 1970s we lived in Blackfeet, Idaho, and I worked at a gourmet restaurant. I was a good cook, but being among all those Potato Kings and their prissy wives was a new experience for me. Once I suggested that the little kids who came to the restaurant, some of whom even had to wear tuxedos, might like a hamburger or a hot dog instead of lobster and steak. The owner's wife told me in no uncertain terms that there would be no more discussion of hamburger at her restaurant.

Anyway, at this fancy restaurant every Tuesday was a smorgasbord. One time we put out a whole fish that must have been three feet long. I was told to make it look nice. I thought, "What am I supposed to do with this?"

I put an apple in its mouth and an olive in its eye. I stood back, looked at it, and it looked wrong. Somehow I knew that that apple belonged in the mouth of a roasted pig. I called Christine, our little German salad cook, and asked her what she thought. She made some sort of cheese log with herb sticks through it. I think the herb may have been rosemary. She stuck that cheese log in the fish's mouth and made it a bridle out of greens, but exactly how she prepared everything, I never knew. It looked very good, whatever it all was.

Soon a customer came back with a request: "We want more of the stuff that's coming out of the fish's mouth." I had no idea exactly what it was, and Christine just made the salads and then went home for the evening. I told them, "I'm sorry, but we have only one per fish. Please come back next time we have a big fish."

❧ Herb Sauce for Fish

½ cup bone marrow or margarine
½ cup Indian lettuce, chopped
1 cup watercress, chopped
1 teaspoon shepherd's purse seeds (or substitute garlic powder)
1 tablespoon lemon juice

Combine the bone marrow, Indian lettuce, watercress, shepherd's purse seeds, and lemon juice in a saucepan and simmer for 20 minutes or until the leaves are tender. Pour over baked or fried fish.

This versatile sauce can also be adapted for red meat. Omit the lemon juice and add 2 bay leaves and 4 tablespoons of water. Simmer an additional 20 minutes, until the leaves are tender enough to bring out the flavor. Add ½ cup chopped onions at this time.

A great herb sauce for fowl can be made the same way, substituting 1 tablespoon of sage for the bay leaves.

Fowl

Quail, sharp-tailed grouse, and prairie chicken were the common wild birds eaten around here. Usually when one was brought in, it was skinned and cleaned, and then boned and boiled. A wild bird and rice made a very good meal. We'd also eat fowl with potatoes or hominy, if we didn't have rice. We'd add a bit of onion if we had it, but we didn't always have it. We'd put just a few leaves of sage in a prairie chicken. Sometimes we'd fry the birds. That was good too.

Pheasant were not so common in the old days, but they were really good when we could get them. My sister-in-law, Mary Ann Hogan, would skin, clean, and gut a pheasant. Then she would cut it in pieces, the way we do chicken, and then she would bread it. She would put the breaded pieces in an oiled bread pan with pieces of onions all over them. Then she would cover it and bake it in the oven for one and a half hours. Salt and pepper went all over it, of course. When the pheasant was nicely browned and almost done, she'd put a little water in the baking pan, cover it tightly again, and stick it back in the oven for maybe another hour. When she took it out, the pheasant was really tender and moist, nice and tasty.

❧ Pheasant and Rice

PHEASANT

1 pheasant, skinned and cleaned
Flour
3/4 cup butter
Salt and pepper
1 onion, finely chopped
2 teaspoons sage
Dried parsley

Split the pheasant in half. Drench the halves with flour. Brown in butter. Season with salt and pepper. Cover and cook the bird for 15 minutes. If desired, add the pheasant liver to the skillet to cook. Add onion and sage. Cover and simmer until the pheasant is tender, approximately 1 1/2 hours. Spoon the pan sauce over the bird. Sprinkle with parsley.

RICE

3 cups wild rice
Water
1/2 cup wild carrots, sliced
3 tablespoons butter
Salt and pepper
Orange slices (optional)

Cook the wild rice covered with water in a 6-quart saucepan. Cook for at least 45 minutes, or until the rice puffs up. Add the wild carrots and butter. Salt and pepper to taste. Arrange on a plate with the pheasant to one side and the wild rice on the other. Garnish with orange slices on each end, if desired.

❧ Spaghetti and Pheasant

Culture Immersion Summer Camp is a place for adults to learn about the culture of the Plains Indians while camping out on the Crow Reservation. This recipe is always a favorite with the participants.

1 pound spaghetti
Water
Olive oil
4 pheasant breasts
2 cups tomato sauce
2 tablespoons garlic, chopped
1 tablespoon dried onion
2 teaspoons basil (or substitute 1 bay leaf)
Salt and pepper

Boil the spaghetti in salted water until it's done (follow the package directions). Drain off the water and sprinkle the noodles with olive oil. Put aside. Cut the pheasant breasts into strips. In a skillet, mix the strips into the tomato sauce seasoned with garlic, dried onion, basil, and salt and pepper. Simmer on the stovetop for 20 minutes. Toss with the spaghetti and serve with a dinner salad and garlic toast made from French bread.

Serves 4.

Wild Turkey: Dagoceshgogeah

Many years ago, even though there are wild turkeys around here, the Crow people had little desire to eat them. We called them "Enemy Bird" because the turkeys would sit on the backs of the horses in a makeshift corral, picking off bugs or whatever. Often one of those turkeys would start to gobble and then the rest would chime in. The horses would get scared, break loose, and run away. It could take hours to round them all up again. So the Crow men called the wild turkey Enemy Bird. "Now we all wait until Thanksgiving to eat enemy bird," says Hank Bull Chief, a Crow elder.

ᶳ Enemy Bird Burgers with Yucca

This recipe is a new use for a common old plant and a healthy alternative to regular burgers. Yucca adds a nice fresh chompiness to the turkey burgers.

Turkey burger patties
Whole-wheat bread
Yucca flowers (about 12 petals, or 2 flowers' worth, per burger)
Your favorite condiments

Grill the turkey burger patties, serve on toasted whole-wheat bread, and top with yucca flowers and your favorite condiments.

Ducks and Geese

I have never seen any Crow hunters go after ducks or geese. I never ate either kind of waterfowl growing up. The first time I tasted duck was at Bill's place, and I was nineteen or twenty then. That was the first time I had goose too. Since then, I have fixed a goose a time or two at Thanksgiving because somebody gave us one. I would roast them in the oven and, well, they were okay, but I really wasn't ever too fond of goose. I guess it's because my people never cared for them as food.

Eggs

Crow people were not any more into eggs than they were interested in ducks and geese, but some folks up north where Bill's people are from consider wild eggs a delicacy. These are some of their stories.

Up north there were these old people. Just before the ducklings were about to hatch, they'd go and get the eggs from the ducks. They'd bring them home, boil water, and throw them in there, these big eggs. They'd cook them for a while. They would take them out after about twenty minutes. They took them out and cooled them off a little. They'd break them, and the embryo was in there. It might even have a feather or two. They removed any feathers and ate the embryo just like that. They thought it was a delicacy. It was only this one couple that did this, but they sure did think it was special.

The same woman up north told me that when her mother was younger, when she was just a kid, they'd go to this island, which is quite a ways from there. They loaded up the wagon and the kids, and they'd all go over there to camp at this lake. And out there was an island in the middle of that lake, where all the ducks went to nest. It was noted for that.

They swam across this lake to that island. They had burlap bags with them. They would collect the eggs in those burlap bags and swim back across and put them in a container. They would drive back, and that's the time when they'd bake a lot with eggs. They ate a lot and baked a lot. They'd have good eating when they'd bring those eggs back.

The lady who told me this story also told me that once her mother even tried bringing back the duck eggs and placing them under her setting hens. She succeeded, and suddenly she had a lot of little ducklings with a hen for a mother. That mother hen kept busy feeding all of them.

When the ducklings got old enough, they wanted to swim. They wanted water. This lady lived not too far from the Milk River. These little ducks would start going over toward the water. The hen would call them back and call them back but then one day they wouldn't listen any longer. So she went with them. The ducklings got into the Milk River. They swam back and forth along the edge, and on the shore the mother hen would run back and forth, clucking, watching her brood swim. And when they'd had enough she would "cluck cluck cluck," and they'd away home to the house of this little lady. They would hang around the hen house again. But it became a habit to swim, so the hen was kept busy. She kept clucking her duckling brood back and forth from the Milk River to the house until the ducks were old enough to fly away.

That was a wonderful story to me.

✿ Stuffed Eggs

This recipe is from my very good friend Emma Lame Bull of the Assiniboine tribe. I have never made it, but it is just like her to mix the flesh of the animal with the eggs, like eating the hen and the baby together.

Many traditional foods were cooked a certain way to make it easier to eat them at a time when nobody had silverware. Cooking the eggs and mixing in the flesh with your fingers would create a dish simple to eat with just the hands.

8 chicken eggs
1 pound ground chicken or turkey, cooked
$1/2$ teaspoon salt
$1/2$ teaspoon pepper
$1/4$ cup butter, softened

Boil the eggs for 5 minutes. Remove them from the heat and set aside to cool, still in the hot water. When they are cool enough to handle, shell the eggs. Split each egg in half lengthwise. Take the yolks out and mash them with the ground chicken or turkey, salt, pepper, and butter. Stuff this mixture back into the egg white halves and serve.

3

Breads

For years and years, meat and wild plants were the main food of the Crow people. Yet, like everybody else, we changed with the times and started adding baked goods and sweet things to our diet as they became available. This chapter talks about breads—which are now a very important part of all Crow feasts—and other simple baked goods. (You'll find the pies and cakes in the fruits section of chapter 1.)

Traditional Bread

The traditional bread food of the Crow people was the wild turnip, but Crows sure took to flour and breads once they had them. Shortening was scarce, and for a long time we didn't have ovens, so the best breads that older Crow people made were those they could bake in the coals or in a skillet over the fire.

✒ Wheel Bread

Pretty Shield always baked her own bread, and most of the time it was wheel bread, ba xaawoo pau gua. Some people call it "bannock." Later she made biscuits, and once in a blue moon she made fry bread, but whenever she had flour, she made wheel bread. Sometimes she would divide the dough into small rounds about the size of pancakes, and these we called coal cakes.

> 5 cups all-purpose flour
> 4 teaspoons baking powder
> 2 teaspoons salt
> 2 cups water

Mix the flour, baking powder, and salt well. Make an indentation in the middle of the mixture and add the water and oil. Mix all together. Knead the dough a little to strengthen it and to keep it from falling apart. Divide it into four sections. Place one section in a 10-inch iron skillet and press it out to fill the whole pan. (You can also divide the dough into 2 sections and use a 12-inch skillet for larger wheels.) Place the skillet on hot coals and bake until the bread is done, about 15 minutes on each side. Repeat with the other pieces. As for most home-baked breads, wheel bread is best eaten warm.

Fry Bread

Bill's mom, Lena Blue Robe, told me that up at Fort Assiniboine, up north around Havre, Montana, close to the Bear Paw Mountains, the trappers would come down and trade with the Indians. Soon the soldiers were trading with the Indians too. The soldiers gave the Indians some iron kettles and skillets to cook with. The soldiers actually taught them what to do with whatever was on hand, like showing them how to sew empty flour sacks into dresses. One time, as Lena told it, the soldiers had salt pork. There was an abundance of salt pork left at the camp because all the soldiers had been transferred back to the main base at Helena to be discharged. They weren't needed at the fort any longer.

And so the soldiers loaded up the salt pork and left a bunch of it at the end of the fort where the Indian encampment was. The dogs went over and kind of smelled around the salt pork, but they didn't touch it. They didn't eat it or even try to. The people went over there, and the men went over too, and they got their sticks and turned the meat upside down and this way and that and said, "There's too much salt on there. Who wants to eat it? It's just inconsumable." And so they left it.

One woman had some flour. The Crow people were all familiar with flour at that time. So she was mixing her flour, and one of the soldiers came along and saw her. She was probably going to make wheel bread or push bread. She was probably going to make that, and he said, "Here's some salt pork that I brought."

She looked at it and shook her head, "No."

But he said, "I'll show you how," and put water in a skillet. Then he trimmed off all the salt and cut the pork into pieces and boiled them. He boiled them in the skillet. Then he threw the water away. Then he boiled it all again and threw the water away. Then he sliced the pork and put it in a skillet and rendered the fat. And after he rendered the fat, he took the bacon out and said, "It's good with bread."

And she said, "Oh, okay. Thank you." And he left. The guy left. And since she had this dough, and the grease in the skillet was hot, she just threw a sample piece of dough into the grease in the skillet. It cooked to a golden brown and rolled around.

She stuck a stick in the fried dough, pulled it out of the skillet, and left it to cool—so the story goes. She turned around and mixed up the rest of her dough, and then she turned back and tested the bread. It tasted good. And so she started putting small amounts in the skillet, so that it would fry like the sample dough. When she took them out, she was very proud of them. So she called the others in, and when they ate the fried salt pork with it, it tasted even better.

So she called the women. She called some women over and said, "Look what I've done."

They tasted the fry bread. They tasted it and said "Mmmmmmm." They were happy with it. So they went and got the flour that they had been given. And they brought it all to this woman and said, "Fix us some bread."

She showed them how to do the bacon, so they did the same. That's how they discovered how to make a new kind of bread using salt pork.

Ba xa woo tom mish a, or Basic Fry Bread

    3 cups sifted flour
    1 1/2 teaspoons salt
    2 1/2 teaspoons baking powder
    1 cup water

Mix the flour, salt, and baking powder together well. Add enough water to make a soft dough. Roll out and cut into pieces of whatever size you prefer. I cut the dough into 4 x 4 inch pieces. Fry in hot grease at 300 to 400 degrees. Cook about 1 minute or so on a side, turning with a long-handled fork. Serve with beef stew. Fry bread is good with juneberry sauce.

Makes about a dozen pieces.

⌇ Fry Bread with Yeast

Fry bread made from yeast dough seems to have a tougher crust. Baking powder bread is more tender, baked or fried.

3 cups sifted flour
2 teaspoons salt
1 package active dry yeast
1 1/2 cups warm water
1/2 cup shortening, melted
2 tablespoons honey or sugar

Mix together the flour, salt, and yeast. Add the warm water, melted shortening, and honey. Mix into a dough. Allow the dough to rise until double in bulk. Roll out and cut into pieces of whatever size you prefer and let rise again. Put the pieces into hot grease and fry at 350 to 400 degrees. Take precautions against the grease splattering. Fry bread is best eaten while hot. Dip it in honey and enjoy.

⌇ No-Rise Fry Bread

This recipe is usually used by vendors selling fry bread at fairs or other gatherings. It is quickly made and fried. That is why it's called "no-rise fry bread."

Follow the recipe for fry bread with yeast but leave the dough a little sticky. Turn the dough out on a floured board and cut into desired pieces. Fry in grease at 300 to 400 degrees until golden brown.

Other Breads

❧ Wild Turnip Bread

While you can eat ehe (wild turnips) as a bread product by themselves (they are very high in carbohydrates), I like breads or little cakes made with a mixture of turnip and wheat flour. Grind dried turnips in a powerful food processor to make turnip flour. (See the wild vegetables section for more information about these fantastic little roots. Remember that they aren't garden turnips at all!)

3 cups all-purpose flour

2 cups wild turnip flour

2 tablespoons or 2 packages yeast

2 teaspoons salt

4 tablespoons shortening

2 ¹/₂ cups warm water

2 to 4 tablespoons sugar (optional)

With a hand whip, gently mix together the flour, turnip flour, yeast, and salt. Add the shortening and warm water (and sugar, if desired). Mix well. Let rise about 45 minutes. Punch down, place in four regular-sized greased loaf pans, and let rise again, another 45 minutes. Bake at 350 degrees for one hour.

❧ Corn Bread

Corn bread is such an important part of the Crow people's diet that I have included two recipes with a couple baking versions. Serve any one of them warm with chili or stew for a simple winter meal.

1 cup stone-ground yellow cornmeal

1 cup unbleached or whole-wheat flour

4 teaspoons baking powder

1/8 teaspoon cream of tartar

¹/₄ cup corn syrup or brown sugar

1 cup milk

1 fresh egg

¹/₄ cup canola oil

Mix together the cornmeal, flour, baking powder, and cream of tartar. Blend in the corn syrup, milk, egg, and oil.

To *bake in an oven*: Put the dough in a greased and floured 9 x 9 inch pan. Bake in 425-degree oven for 20 to 25 minutes.

To *bake in a cast iron skillet over a campfire*: Place the dough in an oiled skillet, cover, and place over hot coals for about 30 minutes, occasionally shifting the dough in a circular motion with a fork until it's done. I sometimes bake the top by removing the lid and propping up the skillet on a forked stick to face the hot coals.

Corn Bread (with sugar)

1 1/4 cups all-purpose flour, sifted
1 cup cornmeal
1/4 cup sugar
2 teaspoons baking powder
1/2 teaspoon salt
1 cup skim milk
1/3 cup vegetable oil
1 egg, beaten

Stir together the flour, cornmeal, sugar, baking powder, and salt. Add the milk, oil, and egg. Mix just until well blended but do not overbeat. Turn the mixture into a greased and floured 8 x 8 inch pan. Bake at 400 degrees for 25 to 30 minutes. Serve warm.

ᎦᎡ Biscuits

Biscuits are an important part of "cowboy cuisine," and all my life the Indians around the Plains have been cowboys, so here's a biscuit recipe.

2 cups flour
2 1/2 teaspoons baking powder
3/4 teaspoon salt
5 tablespoons shortening
3/4 cup milk

Sift together the flour, baking powder, and salt. Cut in the shortening. Add the milk and stir with a fork until a soft dough is formed. Turn out onto a lightly floured board and roll to about 1 inch thick. Cut with a biscuit cutter or form circular patties with your hands and place on a cookie sheet. Bake in a 425-degree oven for 10 to 15 minutes.

Wild berries can be added to biscuit dough. Make certain the berries are strained so they're not too juicy, and sprinkle them onto the flour-butter mixture just before the milk is added.

Makes about 6 good-sized biscuits.

While we were baking and working on this book, Lisa discovered that a warm biscuit with bacon, plum ketchup, and a poached egg makes a different breakfast sandwich.

ᎦᎡ Cornmeal Flapjacks

1 cup cornmeal
3/4 cup wholegrain pastry flour
1 teaspoon baking soda
1 1/4 cup buttermilk (or use regular milk with 1 teaspoon of vinegar added)
1 egg
1 tablespoon vegetable oil

Mix together the cornmeal, flour, baking soda, buttermilk, egg, and oil. Pour out in circles and fry on a hot skillet, turning once.

Makes about 6 good-sized hot cakes.

A TASTE OF HERITAGE FOODS

Hops

According to some people, you can collect hops from hops vines, boil them, and then use the liquid as a wild yeast for yeast bread. Although the vines do grow in Crow country, I have never seen this done.

Sourdough: Baxawewpoah

It was the trappers who brought their sourdough out west here. In the winter, they would sleep with it next to their bodies, so it would not freeze. They had to put their dough starters where it was warm because the yeast organisms are alive. I suppose later on the Indians in their lodges also put their sourdough someplace warm, if they were to have any amount to work with.

The trappers would take a cup of their precious sourdough and mix it with flour. That's about all they had, just flour from the wild, and a cup of it would be a lot. Then they'd make a sourdough wheel bread— just sourdough thrown onto hot rocks or any place that was hot and then covered with leaves to keep the heat in. The Crow word for the sourdough bread that they made, *pajuasa*, simply means, "not like the wheel bread."

Survival Bread

Growing up we didn't have all that much to eat, and we didn't have many food choices. And Pretty Shield had all these grandkids to feed. So, if we had stew or something at noon, in the evening we'd just eat berry sauce and bread. She'd divide up the courses over the day. We'd never have soup and meat and salad and everything all at one meal. Pretty Shield would divide up the day's food, and we'd always have the biggest meal at noon.

My older sister Cerise said that when she was younger, when Goes Ahead was alive and before the Depression, they'd have big meals with many courses. Later, when I was growing up, that never happened. The first of the month, when Pretty Shield received the check from Goes Ahead's pension, she would stock up on all kinds of food. She'd get steak and meat and make jerky or pemmican and store food away. When all that was gone, we'd make do with what we could find. It might be wild plants, or it might be wild meat that one of my brothers brought in, or it might be something really simple and inexpensive, like gravy or fried hardtack. Pretty Shield use to fry hardtack crackers for us quite often. They aren't exactly gourmet, but we grew to like them.

✒ Fried Crackers (Sailor Boy Hardtacks)

Break some Sailor Boy Biscuits (thick crackers, also called hardtack, which were part of the government rations) in half and soak them in ice water for about 3 minutes. Remove them with a strainer-spatula and drain on paper toweling. Transfer the crackers to a baking sheet, cover the cracker with a very generous amount of grease, and bake in a 400-degree oven for about half an hour, or until they are puffed, crisp, and golden brown. They should be dry. Add a little more grease halfway through the baking period, if desired.

A TASTE OF HERITAGE FOODS

PART TWO

Plant Medicines and Healing

A Healing Philosophy

The plants discussed in this book are not meant to be offered as miracle cures. I tell you about them so you can use them as part of a healthy life. A healthy life is more than medicine. A healthy life is built from the inside and includes prevention of illness. To the Indians, food and medicine are largely the same thing. Good foods have healthful properties that are both preventative and healing. If you eat right and exercise, you should stay healthy and not need any "cures."

Of course, sometimes we can't help but get sunburned or bitten or catch a cold from a coworker. These are all excellent times to turn to nature for her wonderful remedies. I hope they will be of some use to you.

Plant medicines have many advantages over chemical medicines. Many of these plants are available free by the side of the road. Everywhere I go I see all this yarrow out there screaming, "A ho, use me."

Most plants have few, if any, side effects, and using plants is usually better for the environment than something bottled. But most people today, they would rather get in their car and go to the store and buy something that's in a pretty bottle and smells good.

After people use the plants, though, they begin to realize what my Grandmother Pretty Shield and so many other Indians knew all along: this stuff works.

This book does not include all the plants used by the Crow people for healing. Medicine men, as they are called, would each have their own special medicines. They would pass down recipes and instructions to their sons or apprentices as carefully guarded secrets. Often the medicines were part of spiritual rituals. Having been raised a Christian in the age of health clinics, I cannot tell you any of these.

What I can tell you are the plant remedies and cures that I learned from Pretty Shield, who had been a powerful and popular midwife. I have also included things I learned from other Crow elders, from my husband Bill's Assiniboine relatives in Fort Belknap, from elders of other tribes we have lived among, and from many modern herbalists and scientists. I've included things I have discovered myself or tried in new ways. Healers come in all shapes and sizes and work in many different ways; here I can share only my way, which is just one way.

Whatever type of healer you become, remember this truth: there can be no healing without heartfelt love and compassion for the person to be healed.

Remember too that our bodies are not all that we have. Our spirits live on long past our flesh, and a healthy spirit is more important than a healthy body.

4

Three Favorite Medicinal Plants

O f all the medicinal plants that grow in Montana, there are three I would not be without. These are yarrow, echinacea, and bear root.

Yarrow: Chibaapooshchishgota
Achillea millefolium
Chipmunk Tail

Chipmunk tail is a "miracle plant." That's what my son, Bill Junior, calls it, and he is skeptical about these kinds of things. *Chibaapooshchishgota*, the Crow word for yarrow, means chipmunk tail. If you look closely at the ferny little lower leaves as it grows out on the prairie, you can see the resemblance to the bushy little tails of chipmunks. This plant has been used for centuries by people all over the world; it seems that you can find these ferny little leaves and the flat, white flower tops wherever you look. It grows in little clumps along the hillsides and trails around here.

Crow people use yarrow, but I learned more about its many uses from the Assiniboine up north and from elders of other tribes that I have lived with. Used on the outside of the body, it is good for easing the pain of bites and stings, healing wounds, soothing burns, and stopping bleeding. Used internally, it helps the urinary tract, is good for the liver, calms the stomach, and helps cleanse the kidneys and prostate.

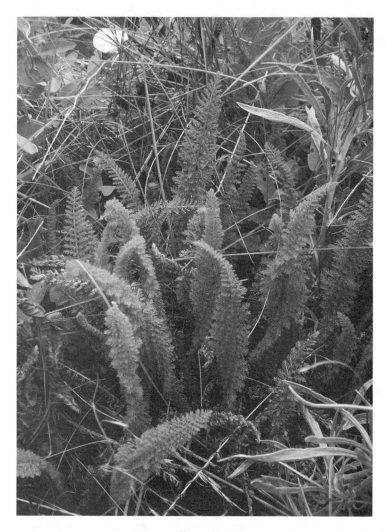

Yarrow

PLANT MEDICINES AND HEALING

Yarrow Used Externally

Sunburns

Awhile back some National Park Service officials spent the whole day out boating in the canyons and on the Big Horn River. By the time they came in, the superintendent was bright, bright red. His skin was so hot and so tight that he couldn't lift his arms. He couldn't even move. He was sensitive to the sun and usually blistered and peeled terribly, so he asked me to try what I use for sunburn on him.

I made him a tea from fresh yarrow leaves and used it as a compress. I rubbed it on his face, shoulders, arms, and neck with a soft cloth. The next day he called and thanked me for it. He never peeled or even blistered, as he was expecting to happen.

Chipmunk tails work for other burns in the same way. I boil the leaves and then soak a dressing in the liquid. I put the saturated dressing on the burn and keep it wrapped up. It seems to heal it quickly and leaves no scars. Yarrow prepared the same way can be tried for skin cancer and pre-cancerous conditions. It should help clear it up.

Cuts

Another time one of my grandsons, Erik, a pharmacist, was helping one of my other grandsons, Billy Three, sand his black Trans-Am sports car. The sander got away from him. It went across his chest and ripped up his clothes and then it dug a big gash down his arm.

Indian Heath Services cleaned him up and wrapped up the wound, but it still hurt. Erik finally came to me for help. I unwrapped his arm, took fresh yarrow leaves and applied them to the cut, wrapped it back up to protect it, and sent him on his way.

As he was working at the pharmacy, his boss noticed this little stem of chipmunk tail sticking out and asked him what in the world it was.

"It's yarrow," replied Erik. "It helps the cut heal and leaves less of a scar, and it has really taken away the pain."

"You mean to tell me that you went to school for six years so you could stick a weed on your arm?" asked his boss.

"Yeah, I guess so," Erik answered.

His boss was tickled that he used "weeds," but Erik was convinced that the yarrow worked.

When they took the dressing off, everyone was surprised that the wound had healed with hardly a scar showing.

Stings and Bites

Usually these days we don't chew on plants and give them to people because of health concerns, but I tell you, there are times when nobody cares about a little spit because something must be done. One time awhile back a man was working on the gas line for the house. He was just finishing up when he was stung. He shouted, "Oh my God, that's a wasp! I'm allergic. I'm going to have to cut my jeans when it swells up and gets too tight."

It was an emergency. I didn't stop and think; I just did something. He pushed his jeans up. I grabbed a piece of chipmunk tail, chewed it a bit, and stuck it to him with a Band-Aid. Then the guy took off driving fast toward Hardin, where the hospital is, about forty-five miles from here.

A few days later we went to pay our gas bill, and we saw him. He called us over and said, "I was anxious, but by the time I got home, my leg didn't feel too tight. I didn't even go to the hospital." When he'd gotten home, he said he took off his jeans, and there was no swelling—just a little red dot where the wasp had stung him.

I've used yarrow myself for a spider bite. One time I was out picking strawberries in my garden. I found this beautiful red strawberry, right under a great big spider web with a giant spider on it. I thought I could just carefully reach under there and sneak that strawberry out without the spider even noticing me. I tried, but that spider was too fast. She bit me.

There were yarrow leaves close by. I grabbed some, wet them with a bit of spittle, and held them to my hand with the bandanna from my hair.

Bill was working close by, so I called to him: "Bill?"

"Yeah?"

"If anything happens to me, it's a spider bite," I told him.

"Okay," he replied, and just kept on working like nothing was wrong.

He was right not to be concerned. I was fine. There was nothing to worry about after I put the chipmunk tail on. That yarrow works wonders.

Yarrow is also useful in the treatment of snakebite. Turn to the snake chapter to learn more about that.

Other Skin Conditions

Very recently, a young woman at church came crying to me because her son, a little boy about two years old, was covered with flaky red patches. He itched everywhere—all over his face, neck, ears, in between his fingers, and on his thighs. Everywhere the skin was red and raw and peeling off. The boy was miserable. The doctor had told the woman that her son must be allergic to dairy or something else. They took dairy out of his diet and still he suffered.

I was thinking about whether or not I could transfer some faith-based healing that an old woman once used on Bill Junior when he was a baby, but I thought, "I might as well apply some yarrow for temporary relief while I consider it." We applied yarrow tea with a piece of damp cheesecloth to all those red patches. I sent them home with some and told the woman to keep applying it to those sores. It wasn't but a few days later when it started to work. She put the yarrow on him, and it started to relieve the itching and the hurting. Then the red sores began to disappear. They all disappeared. After that we gave the boy some dairy foods and then some of the other foods that the doctor thought he might also be allergic to, and it didn't seem to matter. The skin problem cleared up with that yarrow, and it hasn't come back.

I have known for a long time that yarrow works wonders, but it still amazes me when it truly heals right before my eyes. Amazing yarrow. Amazing faith.

Yarrow Used Internally

I learned about drinking yarrow tea from Bill's grandfather, Frank Plume Buck. Every day these old men up at Fort Belknap would drink this greenish liquid. They wouldn't drink quarts of it, just a little bit every day. I was really curious about it and asked Grandpa Plume why he drank it and what it was. Of course, we spoke different Indian languages, and he didn't speak English, so he called his daughter over and asked, "What does my granddaughter want to know now?"

I asked about the yarrow tea. Using Lena, Bill's mother, as a translator, he told me that it was yarrow and that it was good for men's health, especially the urinary tract, kidney, liver, and prostate. He also told her, "My granddaughter wants to know too much." I must have asked too many questions.

After learning from the Assiniboine men that yarrow works internally, I started using it to help people with liver problems. When people have cirrhosis, and the doctor has done all he can, I give them this yarrow. It helps them to come out of it. They leave the hospital and as long as they don't drink alcohol but do keep drinking light yarrow tea, they seem to stay well and live normal lives.

One woman who had horrible cirrhosis left the hospital and lived about three more years once she started taking yarrow. Unfortunately, she started drinking again, and her cirrhosis worsened.

Being a "miracle plant," yarrow is good for more than liver and kidneys. It helps with stomach pains, and it can work for coughs and colds.

One of the doctors at the clinic in Crow Agency had a cough and a dry, sore throat. This doctor came to me one afternoon saying, "Alma, my medicine doesn't work. I wonder if yours will." I made him a pint of yarrow tea, using about four of the leaves in the pint of water. He thanked me and took it home with him. But he didn't drink it. He decided that it smelled too strong or looked too weird or something. His wife, however, was sick and tired of hearing him cough. She couldn't stand the coughing any longer, and he had already tried all of his medicines, so she made him try mine. He drank it all down. His coughing stopped the next day. He was very pleased, and I bet his wife was too.

Try yarrow yourself. It grows almost everywhere, and the results are amazing.

Using Yarrow

The whole yarrow plant—root, leaves, and flowers—can be used, but I like to use the leaves for wounds. For kidney cleansing and such, I would include the flowers too. You can find the "little ferns," the leaves, fresh all summer long. Still, it is good to pick a bunch when you find them and dry them so that you can always have some chipmunk tails on hand.

The traditional way to use yarrow for bites, stings, and scratches is to pick a few large leaves from the base of a yarrow plant. Chew them up well in your mouth. (Warning: yarrow leaves are bitter and taste like medicine.) Once the leaves are wet and soft, press them directly against the scratch, sting, or bite and hold them in place with a clean cloth.

If you don't want to chew the leaves, you can mash them up with a little water until they are wet and soft. Band-Aids and first-aid tape are great modern inventions for holding those chipmunk tails onto the wounds.

For almost every other yarrow remedy, tea is used. To make a strong tea, I use four large leaves per pint of water. For a lighter drink, I use two leaves to the pint. Fresh or dried leaves can be used; it makes no difference. I boil the leaves in the water for ten minutes, then I let it sit and steep while it cools for another twenty minutes. After that, it can be drunk or applied externally with a compress.

Echinacea: Egigeshishibita
Echinacea angustifolia
Black Root, Snake Root, Purple Coneflower

Need an immune booster? Try black root, *egigeshishibita*, which is also often called snake root or purple coneflower in English or even more commonly echinacea, from its scientific Latin name. Like yarrow, black root has many uses, and most tribes of Plains Indians, including the Crow, used it regularly.

The most powerful part of an echinacea plant is the root. Some guys, like Bill, just chew off a bit of the root whenever they think of it. This keeps their immune system strong and helps them if they are bitten by a snake or catch a flu bug. If you don't have a chunk of root close by, or if you can't stand the taste, I recommend taking a little bit of the tincture every day for four weeks. Then leave off of it for four weeks. Then take it again. When you go on and off black root like that, your body doesn't get so used to the echinacea that it quits working. Of course, you can buy echinacea pills at health food stores too. Don't take them all the time either. Be sure to go off them for a few weeks so the plant still has an effect on your body.

Traditional Uses

Black root has long been used for pneumonia and other upper respiratory problems. To use it, make a tea from the root, drench a cloth in it, and put it around the neck. Drink the tea after you're done with the drenching.

The traditional cure for an earache was to burn black root like incense. The healer would catch the smoke in her mouth and blow it into the hurting ear. Then the ear was stuffed to keep the smoke in there.

In the old days the runners, the men who would run from one place to another delivering messages, wouldn't carry any water with them. They just ran from spring to spring or stream to stream. If a runner's mouth started to get dry as he was running along, he would look for some black root. He would take just one petal and chew it. It would draw up the saliva and keep his throat from drying out until he reached the next camp or waterway.

Try it. Take just one petal of echinacea, chew it on the tip of your tongue, and wait for it to tingle.

Chewing a bit of the root (instead of only a petal) will burn your mouth, and then it will make your tongue tingle so much that it will almost go numb. Because of this, echinacea has always been used as a painkiller as well as an immune booster. Chewing on a piece takes the

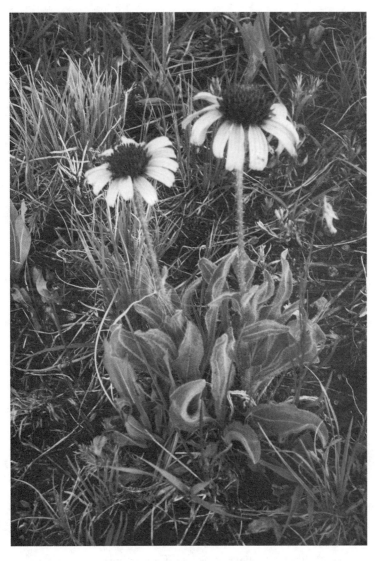

Echinacea

sting out of a toothache. Crow warriors and hunters carried special vials made from a deer joint with a stopper of chokecherry wood. They filled them with powdered echinacea root and tied them to their horses' necks. This location kept the vials from getting caught on trees or in the way between the quiver and the bows, but they were still handy if the warriors or hunters were wounded. They could reach the powdered root and sprinkle a little into the wound. It would stop the bleeding, disinfect the area, deaden the pain, and start healing.

Modern Echinacea Treatments

I have used black root in many more different treatments than Pretty Shield did. I combined what I learned from her and other older Indians with what I have learned from my herbalist friends. Now I make tinctures, which are a new thing, and use them to treat everything from snakebite (see the snake chapter) to toothache to gum cancer. I believe that what with all these new viruses going around, SARS and the like, people really need to keep their immune systems strong. Echinacea is a very useful plant for the world we live in.

I think that echinacea is a wonderful, wonderful root to apply to toothache, especially as a tincture. I had some with me when I was giving a program at a big ranch here in Montana. It's a good thing I had that tincture ready, too, because two archeologists and the Sun Dance leader had tooth trouble at the same time.

I gave them echinacea tincture to apply directly to where they hurt. So they all used it, and they were relieved of their pain immediately. All three were so happy about it. The two archeologists used it until they went home to see their dentists. But the Sun Dance leader, he asked for some more. I gave him some more, but on the second bottle that I gave him I wrote, "Go to your dentist."

He must have. He hasn't come back for any more.

I've used echinacea to treat other mouth problems as well. A girl in Illinois had cankers in her mouth so bad that she couldn't even eat. Poor little thing, it even hurt her to drink water. Her grandpa asked me, "Isn't there anything you can do?"

I just happened to have my tincture with me. I told her I would put it on, but I warned her, "It's gonna hurt. It's gonna burn, but just bear it if you want to get well."

In two days she was well. She was able to eat.

The girl's grandpa kept that bottle of tincture. Before long, he had a toothache. He didn't want to go to the dentist, even though I thought he should. He just kept putting on the tincture, and it would relieve the pain. Then he thought, "Well, if it can stop that much pain, I'm going to use it to pull my own teeth."

Of course I don't recommend this.

He washed whatever instruments he intended to use. Then he jerked his tooth around for a while. He would put a little tincture on it then. He kept doing that; whenever the effect began to wear off, he'd dab a little more tincture on. And he did it. He pulled his own tooth using echinacea tincture. The tincture stopped the bleeding, disinfected his mouth, deadened the pain, and helped the wound to heal.

This man swears by echinacea. He was okay, and so was his granddaughter.

A man closer by, here in Fort Smith, had gum cancer. He chewed tobacco all his life, and his gums were just rotting away. He went to the doctor, who said, "Next time I see you, you may have to go through treatment. This is bad. You have lesions."

So the man met me and asked, "What can you do for me?"

I had just made some echinacea tincture, and I still had the leftover plant pulp in plastic bags in my refrigerator. I though that it might work. I gave him the pulp, and I told him to chew on it instead of chewing tobacco. He didn't want to go through the doctor's treatment, so he tried what I told him.

Meanwhile, this woman who works with him in town was always cleaning up after him in his workshop. She was cleaning up the little piles he leaves on the tables when he chews, and they looked different to her—lighter colored and real woody. She was baffled. She wondered, "What in the world is he chewing now?"

It was black root.

And you know, it worked. I had never seen anyone do this before, but it made sense, and I thought it was worth a try. After three weeks or so of chewing that black root tincture pulp, his sores were all cleared up, and the lesions were gone.

Using Echinacea

You can buy echinacea tincture or capsules, but around here there is black root growing on the hillside if you want to dig it yourself. On these rocky slopes, look for the daisy-shaped flowers with pinkish petals and spiky brown centers. The leaves are stiff and just a little furry. Any given summer, some plants have flowers and some don't, but I don't find much difference in the size of the root underneath. To dig them, use a sharp spade and just pry under the plant until it pops. After you pull up the roots from as deep as you can get them, put the ground back so that you don't leave a hole and so you can't tell anybody has been there.

Once you gather your roots, just wipe them off and let them dry. Chew on a small piece of root every now and then or when you need it. Otherwise, you can make a tincture. Lots of different tincture recipes are out there, and you can follow any of them, but here is one I like, taught to me by an herbalist friend. This one includes alcohol. Different recipes use other liquids for the menstruum, which you might prefer instead.

☙ Echinacea Tincture

> 1 quart echinacea root
> 1/2 cup grain alcohol (like Everclear)
> Water

> Clean roots with clear water. Chop them into half-inch pieces, so that you have about 1 quart of root pieces. Place them in a saucepan with about two inches of water covering the roots. Boil for 4 hours, replenishing the water as it evaporates. Cool. Add the grain alcohol. Pour the mixture into a large dark brown glass bottle. Let the mixture sit for two weeks in a cool, dark place. After that, strain it into a saucepan. Then pour the strained liquid into small dark bottles with dropper caps.

Continue to store in a cool, dark place and use as needed. The tincture is best if used within one year.

For colds, sore throats, and toothaches, I recommend taking the dropper and squirting five drops straight into the mouth and swallowing. For teething babies, I dab a bit of the tincture on a Q-tip and wipe it along the aching gums.

Editor's Note: Commercially available echinacea may be either *Echinacea purpurea* or *Echinacea angustifolia*. The black root found in Crow country, and throughout the short-grass prairie, is *Echinacea angustifolia*, while the purple coneflower plant sold at garden centers is *Echinacea purpurea*. Most evidence suggests that the two species have similar medicinal qualities, yet some herbalists still clamor for wild *Echinacea angustifolia*.

Bear Root: Esa
Lomatium disticum

Of my three favorite medicines, bear root is the most special. Unlike yarrow, which grows everywhere and can be picked anytime, and echinacea, which is not hard to find, bear root is hard to come by. In the old days, only special people—medicine women or shamans—could dig the bear root. They would meditate and pray before they picked it, thanking the Creator for it, and gather it only if they were in the right frame of mind. Because of this, I never dug bear root with Pretty Shield, even though she always had some of it around. It was esteemed as a medicine that was needed almost constantly, and every lodge had some. The lodgekeeper, who we would now call a home-maker, would tie the root up somewhere inside the tipi. Medicines like *esa* were too important to leave on the ground where an animal might get at them.

Before cars and phones and today's conveniences, it was extremely important for healers, especially midwives, to keep their medicines with them and to always be ready. Pretty Shield never knew when somebody was going to have a baby or need her attention. She did not have time to go home and grab her bags and think about it. She had to be ready to just go. So, like other midwives and many lodgekeepers, Pretty Shield always carried a large piece of bear root with her whenever she traveled.

Pretty Shield was a good midwife, one of the best. She helped deliver a lot of babies, including all six of my brothers and sisters and me. She taught me that bear root tea would constrict the womb, push the baby out, relax the mother, and ease her pain. The tea was made from root shavings, about a tablespoon of shavings to a pint of water.

Bear root has many other healing properties that come with prayer. Besides easing delivery, bear root has the power to help with menstrual flow and to ease the pain of women through all stages of their cycles. Tea from bear root shavings also helps alleviate the pain of toothaches and arthritis. Chewing on a spoonful of chopped root pieces and swallowing the juice helps with sore throats and respiratory problems. Bear root can be used in smudging and cleansing too. (Smudging is an aromatherapy type of health help. Some of the root is placed in a little dish and burned, and the smoke is fanned with an eagle feather by the smudger who is helping the ill person.) Bear root even works externally: if you chew on a piece to make a poultice and stick it on the welt from a spider bite, it will help the person who is sick from the bite.

Bears and Bear Root

Like a lot of other Crow words, *esa* does not translate into English. It does not mean "bear root"; it just means what it is. I take *esa* to mean "strength that comes right at you in the face when you take it."

One story that might explain the name "bear root" goes like this. Two boys went on a hunt. It was late in the fall. They went quite a ways from home, looking for game.

All at once a winter storm blew up. It was suddenly cold and snowing. It was a blizzard way up high where they were. They began to realize that they couldn't make out anything with all the blowing snow. They couldn't even see the sun. "Before we get all twisted up worse and lost here, let's seek shelter," they thought. So they looked around and pretty soon they found a cave. They stayed just in the entrance of that cave, but it kept getting colder and colder. Finally they were so cold that they decided to light a fire. One went searching for sticks farther back in the cave. All at once he noticed this big bulk lying there. It was dark, of course, and he couldn't tell exactly what it was, but after he walked around for a minute, he knew it was a great big sleeping bear.

He went out to his friend and made a suggestion. "There's a bear back there. Instead of trying to light a fire in here, let's go back and sleep real close to that big bear and get warm that way." And so they did, and they became warm. Whenever that bear would roll over or start to make some noise, they would jump out of the way and go stand where it couldn't see them. Bears don't have good eyesight, and it was dark, and that bear was mostly asleep. Pretty soon these boys noticed that every time this bear half woke up, it would lick some substance from between its paws, and then it would lick its chops and curl up and go back to sleep. These boys became very curious: just what was the substance that the bear was eating while hibernating? The boys got to daring each other to go find out, until finally one of them took heart and sneaked up and got a little bit of the stuff from around the bear's claws. He sniffed it and tasted it and knew right away that it was *esa*. They decided that *esa* must be what makes the bears go to sleep so comfortably all winter. Maybe that's why they call it bear root.

Oh, and those boys lived to tell about their adventure just fine.

So, I challenge all the scientists out there to study bear root and find out just what the substance is that will make bears sleep so comfortably and to figure out if it works just as well for people.

Bear Root Identification and Use

Esa is in the carrot or parsley family. It has thin little leaves, like the tops of dill, and grows about three feet high. The small white flowers grow in little umbrellas. While you can find it in the summer, it is best picked in the fall. I think the reason Pretty Shield always waited until the fall is that the strength of the plant—the healing power it has in the stem and leaves—had by then been stored away down in the root.

You need to dig fairly far down—a couple feet or so—to get at the root. Then, before you can use it, it needs to be roasted. In the old days, the lodgekeepers would bring in that big black root and throw it on a fire right on the cottonwood coals. They would poke it around with a willow or chokecherry stick until it was roasted on all sides to their satisfaction. They pushed it to one side of the fire and let it cool. After the root cooled off, they would scrape off the outside bark down to the yellowish insides. They would keep that yellowish root whole and chip away little pieces to make tea as they needed them. Just a few chips were put in a pint of water, barely boiled, and then strained.

These days I have heard of people roasting their roots with blow-torches. I don't think that's such a good idea; I wouldn't want any of that gas on roots that I use as medicine. Most of the time I choose to use echinacea or yarrow instead, since they are so much easier to come by, but if I were going to use bear root, I would roast it on a fire of cottonwood or pinewood. Sometimes the old ways really are the best.

Editor's Note: At least two local medicinal species, Lomatium disticum and Ligusticum canbyi have been called "bearroot." Both are considered strong medicine. Because they are members of the very large carrot or parsley family, which contains many poisonous plants, and because wild populations of these long-lived plants are dwindling, they should only be picked with great care.

5

Snakebite

Eyahxasay, snakes, and particularly Eyahxasay awksheeliashyā, snakes that rattle, are a regular part of life in the foothills and plains of south-central Montana. Everyone seems to have a snake story or snakebite cure. I've never been bitten by a snake, but I still have stories and advice to share.

How to Treat Rattlesnake Bites

The old way to treat snakebite was to take some black root (echinacea), chip it into small pieces, boil it, and make a poultice of it. Often the boiled echinacea was mixed with tobacco in the poultice. A healer also hoped that the person who had been bitten had been chewing echinacea regularly to build up his or her immune strength.

Even though using a poultice made from the mashed roots works, I recommend using echinacea tincture in it, a form of the medicine that I have now but my grandmother never did. I wish I never had to learn how to treat a rattlesnake bite, but a few years ago I had a chance to learn firsthand how to treat a bad bite.

Our friend James was out camping. He was picking up a bedroll that he had hung out to dry, and under it was a snake. It reared up and bit him on the calf. He thought it was a harmless bullsnake and didn't think much about it. A few hours later he came to our house. My husband, Bill, looked at the bite; it was bleeding, and it was swelling red. There were two puncture holes. One was bleeding a lot more than the other one, but there were definitely two. James said he felt tingly all over. Bill said, "That was no bullsnake," meaning that it was a rattler.

Right away we offered to take James to the hospital, but he hates hospitals. He put me on the spot and said, "No. Alma, I want you to do it."

Bill and I worked on it immediately. I soaked a cloth in echinacea tincture and applied it to the bite. I also gave him a few drops of the tincture to drink. We asked him to stay and lie down, but he never stays over. So he went. I said a little prayer for him when he was leaving. I knew he wasn't doing well. He was dizzy and woozy. Bill and I both thought he should go to the hospital, but James wouldn't go.

The next day James came back. The swelling was down and the wound looked better. However, he was passing black urine, and he thought that his kidneys must not be working. We offered again to take him to the hospital, but he still wouldn't go. So I tried to figure out what might work for kidneys. I remembered Bill's grandfather used to drink yarrow tea for his urinary tract, and I thought that it might work for James. I made a strong yarrow tea from the leaves and gave him a pint to drink right away. I sent another quart with him and told him to keep drinking it all day and whenever he could at night until his urine was normal.

Then he left. Again I said a little prayer for him because I was afraid. He didn't look well.

Later that night, I said to Bill, "Should we go check on James? He might be lying there dead."

Bill answered, "You've done all you can." But he did come to our home, glad he wasn't dead. By the next day his urine cleared up, and he started feeling better. He never had any problems from the snakebite after that.

How the Crow Learned to Use Black Root for Snakebites

My combination of echinacea tincture and yarrow tea for snakebite may be a new treatment, but using echinacea is a very old method. My stepmother, Lillian Effie Bull Shows Hogan, told me this story about how the Crow learned to use it.

PLANT MEDICINES AND HEALING

One time the enemy was chasing some Crow warriors over near Billings. The Crow warriors were running, running from Cheyennes or Sioux, whoever it was, the enemy. They ran and got quite a ways from them. So these warriors said to each other, "We should stop here and at least rest our horses."

So they stopped for their horses. The enemy was pretty far back, and they were tired too, so they decided to rest awhile and then go on. So they did. Except a rattlesnake bit this one man during the rest hours. His leg started really swelling up big. And he became very, very sick. He told the other guys to go on because the enemy must be coming close. "Go on. Go on ahead and get home and leave me because I'm dying. I'm dying."

His best friend wouldn't leave. "Let's put you on your horse."

But the man with the bite said, "No, I know I'm dying. I'm sick, and I'm hurting so bad that I can't even sit on a horse. I feel it all over. Just leave me. Go on. I'll only slow you down. Go on."

Finally they did. The others left him there to die. They rode off, but this best friend just couldn't leave him lying back there. And so the friend returned. By then the enemy had given up and stopped chasing these warriors. Anyway, the friend had ridden back. As he was riding back to check on his dying friend, he saw a rider coming toward him. The rider was coming right from where they had rested. He scrutinized the rider and realized that it was his friend who had been bitten.

When they met, the friend asked, "How did this happen?"

The man who had been bitten answered that the snake that had bitten him had returned. At least in his hallucinatory state he had seen that same snake, the rattlesnake. The snake said, "Take that plant next to you. Take the root. Chew it. Put it on your bite and be healed."

And so the man reached over and picked this plant. It was black root, echinacea. "Put it on," the snake said. "That will be your medicine to treat snakebites. From now on, your name will be Bull Snake." They called him Bull Snake after that (not meaning a little bullsnake but the chief snake).

So then Bull Snake's medicine became black root, and the Crows have used it to treat snakebite ever since.

Other Ways to Treat Snakebites and Other Bites

My son Bill Junior worked one summer on a road crew. It was hard, hot work, and they saw lots of snakes. A rattler was rearing up to strike a man when the man spit his chewing tobacco straight into the snake's mouth. The snake stopped suddenly and died on the spot.

The men were all amazed and wondered if what they had seen was just a fluke or if tobacco juice really worked to kill rattlesnakes. The next time they saw a snake, they caught it and spit chew into its mouth. That one died too, immediately. They swear that it works.

Try sprinkling tobacco on the ground around your camp. It may keep the snakes away.

My grandmother told me of another way to cure snakebite. Once there was a lady who was picking plums off the ground. She was in a big hurry and picking them up fast, so she could get just as many as she could. She didn't stop and see that there was a snake among the leaves on the ground. (Watch out when you pick plums because snakes really do like plum leaves. Pretty Shield always told us to be careful. She told us to beat around with a stick before we picked plums.)

The snake bit the lady. It bit her. My grandma's mother took some of the plum leaves and crushed them and put them on the bite as a poultice. The leaves drew a lot of the venom out, and the swelling went down. The woman got well, but she always had nervous actions afterward. They say that after she was bitten, her tongue went in and out of her mouth real fast. And all the rest of her life, when she walked she would wave back and forth a little. Grandma said that snake must have left part of himself in her along with the venom.

Snake Avoidance

Of course the best cure for snakebite is not to get bitten at all. I always go out carrying a big stick and making a lot of noise, so they stay away. It seems to work. I haven't ever been bitten.

Bill's grandma, One Woman, was superstitious about keeping snakes away. She taught Lena that when you keep rattlesnake rattles around the house, other snakes will make their way over to your house.

Now Bill's uncle used to kill snakes and keep their rattles. One Woman told us all, "My son-in-law, he should get rid of those rattles. I dreamed the other night that there were snakes all around looking our way. It's because he has kept those rattles." One Woman's daughter, Blue Robe, turned and looked right at him, "Get rid of them!"

And he did, not because he believed the superstition but because he had so much respect for One Woman. I don't know if his disposing of the rattles is the reason, but we never did have any snakes around that house after that.

Pretty Shield had a very simple method for keeping snakes away. She would just tell the snakes, "This is my path. This is where I harvest. You need to stay away from my grandchildren and me. Your place is out there." She'd point out into the sagebrush. "Your place is out there. Go."

I was just a little girl at the time, and I thought that the snakes obeyed Grandma just the way I obeyed her. The rattlesnakes stayed away. They listened.

I know now that snakes don't have ears, so that scientifically, they couldn't have been listening to Grandma, but I still think they knew what she said. She was a very powerful woman.

6

More Medicinal Plants

Along with my three favorite plants and those used to treat snake-bite, I have used a whole range of medicinal plants that grow here on the plains and in the mountains of Montana. The plants listed in this section show the variety of what I have used, but it does not include many wild medicinal plants that you may have heard of. Some of the plants I didn't include, like clover and osha, I have no personal experience with. People tell me that they work, but I have never used them myself. Other plants are toxic medicines, and I don't mess with them. There were medicine men who worked with lupine (*Lupinus* species), foxglove (*Digitalis* species), baneberries (*Actea* species), and nightshade (*Solanum* species), but I don't know exactly how they used these poisonous plants. Since giving the wrong amount can really hurt someone, I stay away from them. I don't want to be trusted with something unless I'm really sure of it. I recommend that you do the same. Never swallow anything unless you know what it is. Pick plants with somebody who is an expert for your area. Learn to identify the poisonous plants growing in your region.

These plants are arranged alphabetically by their common name in English.

Arrowleaf Balsamroot: Augaurashkose see ga
Balsamorrhiza sagittata

Every spring the yellow flowers of arrowleaf balsamroot cover the hills just up from our house. The yellow daisy-like flowers sticking out of big clumps of pale green, arrow-shaped leaves are a great sight after a long winter. Arrowleaf balsamroot is good for "sores that cannot be healed," which I take to include staph infections, syphilis, and cancer. The one time I saw it used, the person pulverized the root in some water, saturated a thin buckskin with the medicinal water, and dressed the wound with that buckskin. The patient then kept his whole leg, dressed wound and all, out in the sun. He even kept it in the sun after they took the dressing off. This treatment seemed to heal his "wound that could not heal."

If I were using arrowleaf balsamroot today, I would suggest cooking the root in a little water, pulverizing it, and packing a wound with some cheesecloth soaked in the water. With all we know about skin cancer, I wouldn't put the wound out there in the sun for too long. For the more adventurous, I might suggest mixing the pulverized root with clean earth, the way that Pretty Shield used to make medicinal mud packs, and applying the mud-root mixture right on the wound.

The roots and leaves of arrowleaf balsamroot are also edible, but they are more of a survival food than a wild mountain delicacy.

Burdock Root
Arctium minus

I gave a chopped up burdock root to a young man who was concerned about his grandfather. His grandfather had gallstones and was unable to eat at all. Whenever he took a bite of any kind of food, he became sick. The young man imagined that his grandfather was starving, and the doctors couldn't operate because of the man's age and weakened condition. I instructed him to take the burdock root and make tea, strong, and give it to his ailing grandfather. So he did. The report after a few days was good; those stones must have passed or dissolved. In either case, his pain went away and he lived about five more years, and he had been eighty already.

I know that to most people burdock is just an annoying weed. It is not even a plant native to this continent. Still, weeds can work wonders sometimes. Elders and some herbalists tell me that the burdock root is also good for arthritis and rheumatism. The whole plant is edible and has a high mineral content.

Cedar Berry: Bage eli gee chi bagua
Juniperus horizontalis
Creeping Juniper

Feel a headache coming on and don't have any willow bark around? Eat four or five cedar berries. It should clear it right up. The little berries from the cedar that creeps low to the ground are also good for sore throats and lung congestion. Of course junipers and cedars are widely used for incense and these days they are common for Christmas decorations.

Editor's Note: Junipers and cedars regularly cause confusion, and not just because there are more Crow words for them than English words. A huge range of unrelated plants are commonly called cedars. The cedar berries referred to here are from the creeping juniper, *Juniperus horizontalis*.

Cherries
Prunus species

Cherries are good for taking away the pain caused by gout. I have a gouty heel, and sometimes it hurts so badly that I can hardly stand. But if I drink lots of water and eat cherries, I can walk and bend my ankle without pain.

Of course, chokecherries (*Prunus virginiana*) were used traditionally, but I find that if I eat even bing cherries, they have the same healing effect.

Corn (Silk): Xoxashegia
Zea mays

The silk from an ear of corn will help you if your feet or joints are swollen. Dry corn silk in the oven, make a quart of tea from it, and drink the liquid. You don't need to drink the quart all at once. Keep drinking a little throughout the day and night until the quart is gone, and your swelling should go down. It must be a diuretic.

I learned how to use corn silk from a Chinese woman, even though corn is a plant native to America. She also taught me that you could use the same corn silk three times for tea if you dry it out between uses. I have prepared and administered this treatment to a lady with swollen ankles with great results.

Dandelion
Taraxacum officinalis

Dandelion is another plant from Europe that most people see only as a weed, but, like burdock, it has its uses.

According to a Crow folk remedy, the milky sap from a dandelion stem will cure warts if you rub it on the wart several times a day. I have never tried it, but they say it works, and it couldn't hurt you.

Bill's aunt, Katy Birch, had diabetes. She made a broth of dandelion roots, stewing them in hot water with sorrel and the yolk of an egg. Taken daily for some months, this really seemed to help her with the diabetes. I have also heard that dandelion root broth helps with liver problems, mostly in men. It seems to work something like yarrow and helps with the liver, kidneys, and urinary tract. Generally though, we think of dandelion as a little extra food, and you can read more about it in the wild greens section in chapter 1.

Flax: Esshogebalia
Linum species

Blue flax (*Linum lewisii*) grows wild here, and I've heard of it being used in the old days. Still, I have never seen anyone use the wild plant. I buy flaxseed oil, made from cultivated plants, from the health food store for modern uses. It's good for dry coughs, and a poultice made with the oil will calm headaches and earaches. I also tried using flaxseed oil once in a while in my biscuits. It doesn't work as well as canola oil, but trying it doesn't hurt anything.

Grapes: Dax bee chay ish ta shay
Vitus species

Wild grapes are a favorite food around here, but they can also be used for healing. Grapes are good for the eyes. Dip a cloth in the cool liq-

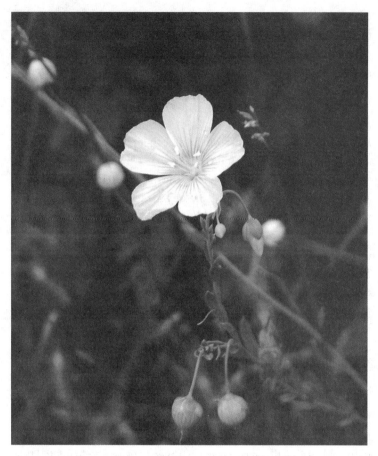

Flax

uid made from crushed grapes and place it over your closed eyes. The grape juice helps with the circulation in the eyes and brings up the blood, I believe. It helps you to see better and helps with the trouble of twitching eyes.

Grapes, dried with the seeds and all, are also taken for tumors and for cleansing the blood. It's good tonic for what the old ones called "ailments that don't heal," which I always take to mean cancer. It has helped patients with tumors and may have even shrunk them. Nowadays I recommend people take grape seed extract or drink lots of Concord grape juice if they don't have wild grapes.

Hawthorn: Beelee chi sha yeah
Crataegus species

Hawthorn is a very special food and a special medicine. As for collecting bear root, people meditated before they picked the fruits from these beautiful trees. Women would go together to pick the fruits at the end of the summer. They would set down their little pads and sit down and pray before they started picking. I saw women do that when I went picking with Pretty Shield, but because I was a child, I didn't actually know what they were doing. I just played around until they were ready to pick, and then I'd go help them.

I learned later on from Hank Bull Chief that the women had been meditating and telling the Creator, "Thank you. Thank you for this that we are taking. Thank you for blessing us with good health with this food. We pray that you will protect us from any bad effects that would be surrounding it. Thank you for your provisions. Thank you for feeling sorry for us, for loving us so much that you provide this food."

Then they'd say thank you very much again and sit for a while. They'd wait for each other to finish this meditation, this talk or prayer. When everybody got done they'd all say, "A ho!" (thank you!). Then they'd stand up and wash their faces in the stream and freshen up to go at the picking. But before they'd pick they'd always say, "*dis w ba desh wa week.*" That means, "Hawthorn, I will prepare a pair of moccasins for you."

As a child I wondered, "Why do they say that when a hawthorn has no feet? Where is the tree going to put the moccasins?"

After I grew older I began to see the reason behind it. You must give as well as take. The women figured that in promising to give back, they allowed the tree to grow more. Trees grow from the root, the feet of the tree. "Making moccasins," dressing the roots, is a way of taking care of the tree. The women were also promising not to pull it out by the roots or prevent it from bearing again and again.

Once they are picked, hawthorn berries (also called haws) are good food, although not the best. Pretty Shield had us eat them because we needed food, but she also knew that hawthorn was a powerful plant. The berries are more than just nourishment. They are good for the heart, for "pushing blood," for chest pains, for upper respiratory complaints, and they are good for the bowels.

Crows think hawthorn breaks apart clots in the blood veins, ta de way. It also strengthens the muscles of the heart. For palpitating hearts, hawthorn acts as a stabilizer, and it helps the heart beat at the right rhythm.

To use hawthorn as medicine, eat the berries. If I wanted to treat myself, I'd eat a handful every day. You can also cook hawthorn. Make a hawthorn sauce, and don't mix anything with it. Take that sauce, about a tablespoonful every three hours, and drink a substantial amount of water. Sometimes the hawthorn bark is also used but not nearly as often as the berries.

If you eat hawthorn as a regular food and eat it fast, say as a jam on bread, most of it will go right through you and not do you any medicinal good. Eat hawthorn plain (no sugar and spices) and slowly when you want to take it for heart medicine.

My son-in-law's mother had heart trouble a few years back. The doctors informed her children that she might not come out of surgery but that surgery was her only chance. They told them to prepare for her to go, but that she might make it.

My son-in-law called me and said it was because of her weak heart that she might not be able to make it. It came to me immediately to give her huge doses of hawthorn, if the doctor was willing. The doctor said it was okay, go ahead.

For the two weeks before surgery, she took megadoses of hawthorn pills, the kind you can buy any day at a health-food store.

When she went into surgery, nobody knew what would happen. They didn't know whether the hawthorn would work or not. But she survived the procedure and afterward the doctor said, "It was amazing to me. The muscles of her heart were so strong. Nothing at all like the weakness we found just a few weeks before."

So then they reminded him, of course, that hawthorn was what she was taking. The doctor said, "Hawthorn. That's good to know. We might need to follow up on that."

That was a few years ago. She lived. She recovered fully. She even went to Hawaii. She's eighty-three now or somewhere in there. They say that she's just doing fine with that heart. She's still taking hawthorn, and she won't be without it.

I went to Washington DC, a few years back. After I got there, on about the second day, this man came over to me and said, "My son just called me, and he has MS. He's a musician. It just breaks his heart that this MS has taken its toll. He can't play, and he's just devastated. His music is his livelihood."

I told him to have him take hawthorn, not because he has a problem with his heart but because I know that it strengthens muscles. I instructed him to take hawthorn at the highest strength sold and to follow the directions on the bottle. And so he did.

The next month I was in Washington DC again. This same man rushed over to me and said, "I want my whole family to meet you. I want to take them to Montana to meet you because of what you have done for my son. He started taking that hawthorn, and now he's playing again. A month later, and he's back on the job. Thank you very much." The man's son continues to take hawthorn.

And that's the testimony from people I know whom I've given hawthorn to. In fact, I use hawthorn myself—not because I'm ailing but for prevention perhaps.

Horsetail: Auxbawlax ecoosua
Equisetum species
Joint Weed, Ghost Pipe

Crow runners used to place the ferny bases of horsetail in their moccasins to prevent leg cramps, I have been told. I have also heard that old Crows used horsetail to help people breathe better. I also believe it stabilizes blood pressure.

Juneberry: Bacu:wu:lete
Amelanchier alnifolia
Serviceberry, Sarviceberry, Saskatoon, Shad Bush

Juneberries help the eyes. Eating them is good for the eyes, and eye drops can be made from the strained liquid left after juneberries have been boiled.

Upset stomachs can also be brought under control by eating juneberries. Of course, juneberries taste so good that kids sometimes eat too many and upset their stomachs. You can read the tempting recipes for juneberries in the fruits section of chapter 1.

Kinnikinnick: Obeezia
Arctostaphylos uva-ursi
Bearberry

At one of my demonstrations, a boy got up and asked if he could say something. At the time, I was talking about kinnikinnick (*Arctostaphylos uva-ursi*) and how it can be used for food and in pipe mixtures.

I thought, "This ought to be interesting," and told him to go ahead.

He said, "I had asthma so bad that I couldn't hardly breathe anymore, and the doctors couldn't do any more for me. I was in bad shape. Then I went to this medicine man. He took some kinnikinnick, with shavings of the bark and the berries. Nothing mixed with it, just the kinnikinnick. And he made a tea."

He drank that tea, the boy said, and it worked. It checked his asthma. He just wanted to stand up and give his testimonial that day.

Inhaling the smoke also seems to open the sinuses.

Lichen: A wa ga chilua
Xanthopcimelia chlorchroa

My stepmother, Lillian, had a great uncle who was a chief of a group of Crows that settled in Red Lodge, Montana. He was one of the sub-chiefs, the chief of that group. They looked for a place where there was plenty of wood, plenty of game, and plenty of water: a good place to camp. They found it near Red Lodge, so they settled there.

One day during the time when it gets frosty at night but still melts during the day, a whole string of wagons came over the hill. It was a wagon train. It was a train of immigrants that were going to set-tle in this country. They were traveling west, but they were afraid to go any farther because of the cold coming on. They needed to settle down and winter someplace. They sent their messengers out, and the chief's messengers also went over to meet them. Everything was ex-plained, mostly by sign language. The messengers came back and told the chief that the train of people wanted to settle someplace close by. If he would allow them to camp for the winter, they'd be very grateful. Then, in the spring when the snow was gone, they'd move on west.

The chief got together his men, the elders, and they talked about it. They decided the settlers should camp a ways from them but where they were still visible. The chief told the settlers, "There's a good camping place over there. You should find lots of wood and lots of game. You'll do well there until you're ready to move on." So the set-tlers went there, and they made themselves cozy. And the Indians were cozy in their camp too. Everybody got along fine. Each camp had their own thing going, and they didn't bother one another.

One day, though, the chief heard a cry, like a mourning cry, from the settlers' place. He said, "Go and check it out to see if they are hav-ing a bad time over there. Have the women fix some food and take it over there, as we do when one is lost." And so they did.

They went over there and came back and said that a little child had died.

After they came back, another cry went up. More children were get-ting sick, and now they were dying.

These messengers must have brought the bug back because soon after the chief's children—a boy about twelve years old and a girl about ten—they got sick. They got sicker and sicker. The Crows tried all the different medicines that they had on hand. The medicines relieved the children's sickness for a little bit, but it would never go away. The children were getting worse. Their necks were swollen. Their ears hurt. Their throats seemed swollen. They labored in their breathing. So the chief said, "This thing is something I don't recognize. I am going to go fast and see if help will come to me to treat these people and my people."

The chief went out. He grabbed his robe and told his wife, "Keep the fire going and keep some water hot." And so he went. He took his robe, and he went out to fast, far away from camp.

He picked a place and there he stayed for four days. On the fourth day, with no answers, he decided that no help was coming to him. So he picked up his robe and turned around to go and at that moment he saw all this lichen, ground lichen. The ground was completely covered with it. He said, "I didn't see this when I came, and now it's here. This must be my help."

So he took a bunch of the lichen and put it in the arm of his robe and took it home. He told his wife to hurry up and make some tea and give it to the children. His wife told him that she thought the little girl was already dead, and in the meantime other children from both camps had gone.

The chief knelt by the little girl, and he worked on her and tried to bring her back to breathing. In the meantime, his wife made some tea and dripped it into the mouth of his little girl. They kept putting it in there and putting it in there until she began to cough. She was coming out of it, so they helped her sit up. She coughed scabby stuff out of her throat, and she began to breathe.

The chief told his wife, "Make some more of this tea and give it to the girl. Make the boy take it too." His kids got better after this. Their fever and swelling went down, and they felt better.

So he sent a messenger over to the settlers' place to tell them to use

PLANT MEDICINES AND HEALING

the lichen, and he told his own people to go and pick the lichen and to use it for their own children when they became sick. The messengers went and told everyone. They hurried and picked the lichen and did as they were told and gave it to their children. That's what healed them. It cured them of this disease.

Both the settlers and Crow people were very happy and joyful. They all loved their children. They had a lot in common. No doubt they had some exchanges of food and some celebrating.

Judging from the symptoms, I think it was diphtheria.

And that's how a lichen, *Xanthopcimelia chlorchroa*, a foliose lichen that grows on the rocks or rocky ground around here, came to be used for sore throats, even to this day. My sister Mary Elizabeth came out here and said, "I see you've got some ground lichen." She picked some and chewed it because she had a bit of a sore throat. As she was chewing it, I remembered that it was her own mother who told us the story of the chief and the lichen.

They were very helpful toward one another in those days. They had to be.

Milkweed: Cetizbaxupe
Asclepias speciosa

Lots of old people use the milky sap of milkweed for swollen joints and arthritic ailments.

One man's knee was so bad that he couldn't walk. He was trying to get around on crutches when he ran into a very old Indian lady. She asked what was wrong. He showed her the knee that was so swollen and red and hurting. She went and picked some milkweed and brought back the milky part of it. She mixed it with a little water, so that it would be easy to take down. He took it. He took it for four days, about one-half cup per day.

Now he's walking about. There's nothing wrong with his knees.

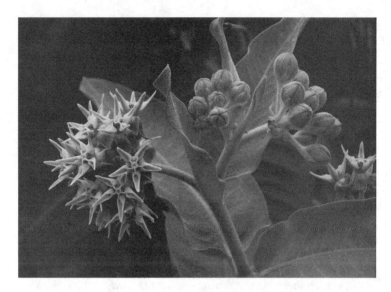

Showy milkweed

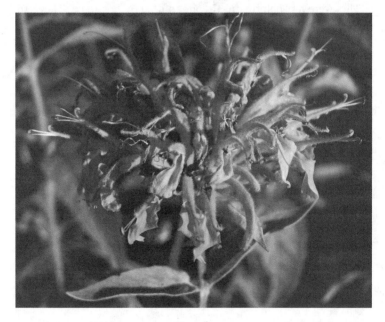

Monarda

PLANT MEDICINES AND HEALING

Mint: Shushue
Mentha arvensis

While mint is used mainly to make an enjoyable tea and to flavor foods, it also has healing properties.

Mint is good for calming flatulence, settling the stomach, and freshening the breath. Mint has a way of stimulating the bladder. It's not quite as healing as cranberry juice, but the effect is similar. Mint is calming, cooling, and good for the stomach. Even if you drink mint tea hot, it will cool you inside.

Wet mint placed in cheesecloth and pressed around both temples and across the eyebrows is a good remedy for a headache.

Mint should not be given to a pregnant woman, as it may cause a miscarriage.

Monarda: Aw wa xom bilish bi baba
Monarda fistulosa
Bee Balm, Mountain Mint

Besides making a great tea, *Aw wa xom bilish bi baba*, monarda, has a lot of oils, so it makes a good poultice. Use it on rashes and red skin because it is not too strong.

Monarda tea is soothing to me. I drink it for a relaxing effect. It quiets the stomach and calms one down. It also seems to stabilize diabetic upsets in people.

Sphagnum Moss: Bee ma ga sut che
Sphagnum species

A little bit of sphagnum moss makes a good poultice for sores and wounds. A small amount grows around here (there's a little patch right next to my pond), but greater amounts grow in western Montana and other places with a lot of moisture. The moss makes a good healing poultice for open sores. The plant is very absorbent, so putting it in the cradle with a baby will soak up the moisture and help keep the baby dry. Moss can also be dried and saved for future use.

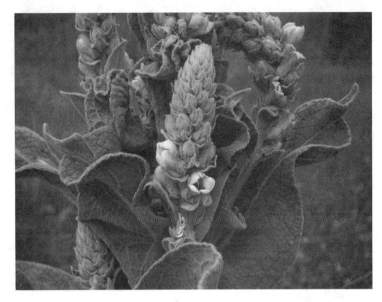

Mullein

Mullein: Aubeesay
Verbascum thapsus

Mullein, a plant with large, soft leaves, is another common roadside weed that can be put to good use. The leaves were used for hygienic purposes (I hear some call it "farmers' toilet paper"), including during menstrual cycles and for lining babies' cradles. Lactating women crushed the leaves, moistened them a little, and laid them on their breasts for better flow and more milk for the baby. I've heard that mullein is also effective in treating virus-type pneumonia. Beyond all this, mullein leaves are also edible, if they are boiled twice and you are really hungry. I chewed one once, and it was not very good, but I ate it.

Nettles: Babaliatocha
Urtica dioica

Stinging nettles seem like a horrible weed. They are very painful to handle or walk through, but once you realize how useful they are, you might actually want nettles growing in your yard.

The nettles can be eaten (if you boil the leaves twice, dumping out the water after the first time) and are very good for you, high in minerals. Stinging nettles taken internally help a lot of allergy attacks. Drink a tea made from the leaves or take the capsules you can now get in health-food stores.

Growing up, I never saw anyone drink nettle tea, but they did whip themselves with the plants during sweats. It works like this: if someone has arthritis or joint problems, tie stinging nettles into a bundle, and then switch the person with them. It will relieve their pain. Each of the little stingers is like a small shot of histamine. I guess the person will start itching instead of hurting. It doesn't sound fun to me, but I understand that it works.

I have never done it myself, but I did tell a priest to do it once. He said it helped.

More recently, stinging nettle capsules were taken by my son, Ted Kills In The Fog, for a terrible attack of pollen allergies this past spring. His eyes were red and watering and his sinuses were full. After taking the nettle capsule the second day all was A-Okay.

Oregon Grape: Away daubish bagua
Mahonia repens
Creeping Mahonia, Grape Holly

Oregon grape bears little purple grapelike fruits late in the season. Pick them when they are dark and sweet, and you can eat them just like grapes.

The roots of a good, healthy specimen can be crushed and used for growths on the neck. They are good for tumors and cysts, even those that you can't see, such as in the brain. I have seen people eat these grapes for inward healing.

Ponderosa Pine: Ba geeah
Pinus ponderosa

A story I've heard is of an old lady from Rocky Boy (in northern Montana). They say she had the remedy for cancer. She treated a lady with cancer, and she was healed. Unfortunately, the healer refused to tell her secret remedy to anyone to the day she died. She took it with her. Others thought that her secret was some pine needles. What kind of needles is a guess, but I'd guess ponderosa pine. I'd like to see some scientist study the pines and see if we can't better fight this awful disease.

Plantain: Begeelish aubalay
Plantago virginicum

The leaves of the little weed called plantain work well for packing cuts and open sores. Look around your yard. You probably have this plant growing right by your house. Across the Big Horn River from here is a ranch called Grape Vine. A lady friend of ours, a real horse lover, worked there. She came to our home one day very upset because her filly, almost two years old, had been cut by barbed wire on the right hind leg. It was a bad gash. The horse wouldn't allow anyone to get near its backside. The leg trembled, hurting bad. The cowboys at the ranch had decided to put the filly out of its misery, but my friend couldn't stand the idea.

So I went with my friend and poured some powdered willoprine (the aspirin-like substance from willow that you can buy at a health-food store) into the horse's feed. My friend fed her filly, and it ate. Twenty minutes or so later, I went into the stall, and the horse allowed me to brush her hips with my hand. I plucked some plantain growing right there and made a poultice as I stroked her. I tied it on the wound and instructed my friend to keep doing the same thing, changing the dressing often.

By the next day the horse was able to walk very slowly and carefully. The wound kept healing, and before long they were able to transfer that horse down to a ranch in Wyoming. She recuperated, grew up with only a slight limp, and later gave birth to a healthy foal of her own. That is the success story of healing a wounded horse with a plantain poultice.

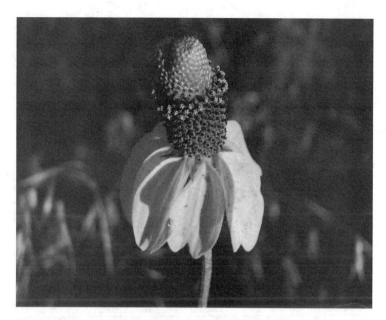

Prairie coneflower

Prairie Coneflower and Purple Prairie Clover:
A wa chu geba a ba lee shee la
Ratibida columnifera and *Dalea purpurea*

Prairie coneflower (also called Mexican hat) and purple prairie clover flowers were made into teas and used for chest and respiratory problems. The prairie coneflower tea tastes good, and I have a friend here in Fort Smith who drinks it as a social tea. Visit her in the mornings, and she'll likely serve you prairie coneflower tea along with delicious wild plum cake.

Sage: Esushgexuwa
Artemesia species

One time when I was a young girl, I was running to my uncle's place because somebody was trying to beat me up. I'm sure I deserved it,

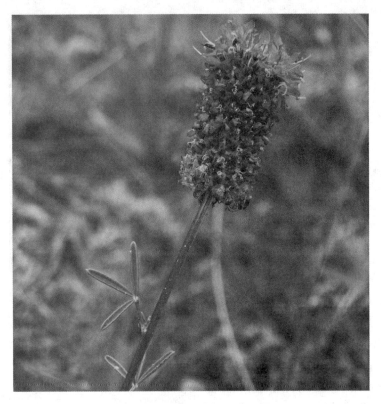

Purple prairie clover

but I wasn't going to let her catch me. I had almost gotten away, but just as I was reaching for the doorknob, she caught me from behind. I fell, smacking my nose hard against the doorknob.

The blood wouldn't stop, and my nose was broken. Herbert Old Bear took me and stuffed sage into my nose. Then he stuck me underneath a canvas and started burning a sweet pine smudge.

The bleeding stopped, and I can still breathe, so it must have worked well.

That was my first experience with sage used for healing. Since then I have learned to use the many different types of sage (*Artemesia*) that grow around here. Big sage (sage brush, *Artemesia tridentata*), silver

PLANT MEDICINES AND HEALING

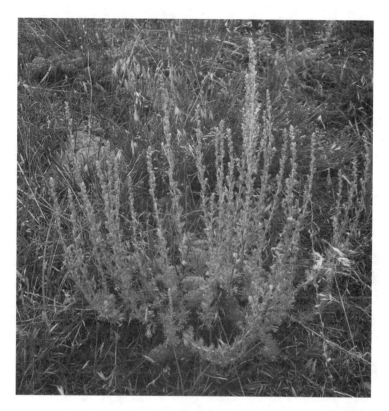

Sage

sage (sweet sage, *Artemesia ludoviciana*), and fringed sage (*Artemesia frigida*) are the most common, and all three have a healing effect on infections. They can help stop bleeding externally and internally, although they are not often used internally because sage can have an adverse effect on the liver.

When men, especially warriors, felt that they had too much blood, they bled themselves. They would make a cut in their arm and drain out some blood. Then they would stop the bleeding by curling up their arm and putting sage in the crook on top of the cut. I saw my father do this once, and he seemed to think it really helped him.

While we were out hunting for turnips while working on this book,

Lisa's friend Tracy was stung by a sweat wasp. Immediately her leg turned red surrounding the bite, and she began to get welts. There was no yarrow or echinacea close by, so I grabbed some sage and had her chew the leaves and stick them right over the bite. She held them there and then did it once more on our way home. By the time we arrived, the sting didn't itch any more, and we couldn't even find the spot where she had been stung.

Besides for stopping bleeding and treating small wounds, sage is often used for cleaning and clearing up bad smells. I figured that the two effects together would be perfect for my friend who had lupus. She was bleeding from the inside. Every time she bled, you could smell it. My grandson, who was very young at the time, loved to play with her but would come home and ask why she smelled so bad.

I gave her wormwood sage (*Artemesia ludoviciana* that has gone to seed) in tea form. I didn't know if I was doing anything right, but I had to try something. I made her a tea and gave a pint to her, to be taken over four days, which is our way. The sage helped check the bleeding, helped balance her blood levels, and sure made her smell better.

Sage doesn't work just on people. It can be very effective for animals too. Once I went into a restaurant to have a spot of tea when a young lady came up to me and very sadly told me about her ferret. It seems the ferret was losing hair, becoming bare and ugly, and its teeth had become loose. Rather apologetically, she asked if I knew anything that might help her poor ferret. I sent her the leaves of silver sage and told her how to administer them. She was to boil the sage in water for ten to fifteen minutes, let it cool, and then apply the liquid to the affected areas and rub it on the ferret's gums and mouth.

Less than three weeks later that ferret had all its hair back—a lush, full coat—and its teeth were stronger. I rejoiced with the young woman and her pet.

Editors Note: "Sage" often refers to garden sage (*Salvia officinalis*) and other species of Salvia in the mint family as well as sagebrush (*Artemisia tridentata*) and the many other species of *Artemisia* that are in the daisy family. *Salvia* and *Artemisia* have a similar fragrance, and both can be gray leafed, but the similarities end there. Here we are refer-

PLANT MEDICINES AND HEALING

ring to *Artemesia* species, not *Salvia*. "Wormwood" most often refers to the European plant *Artemesia absininthe*, but, as many species of *Artemesia* are used against intestinal worms, this common name has come to be applied more generally. Here, the term wormwood is used to distinguish the flowering and fruiting stalks of *Artemesia ludoviciana* from those stalks with only broad flat leaves, called silver sage.

Saw Grass

Spartina pectinata

Prairie Cord Grass

Saw grass has very sharp blades, and it grows way out on the prairie. Bill's father, Babe Snell, told me once about a medicine man called Medicine Boy who cut out somebody's cataracts with it. Then he washed out the eye, put a bandanna over it, and told the patient not to open his eye to light for quite awhile. That man suffered. The surgery and healing were really painful for him. But after he took the bandage off, he saw really well.

That was the only time I've ever known of anyone to take cataracts out with grass. I don't recommend that you try it at home.

Snowberry: Bitdaja

Symphoricarpus occidentalis

When I was growing up, Pretty Shield forbade me to eat the white berries on the snowberry bushes because they are toxic.

Years later, Hank Bull Chief, who is a Crow elder, told me that his father would take five of them, and they really cleared his head. He treats sinus problems and head colds with them.

In one of my presentations at the Little Bighorn Battlefield Site, I mentioned that snowberries were used this way. A woman, a tourist in the audience, came up to me at the lunch break and asked for some snowberries. I refused, telling her that my grandmother had told me that they were poisonous, that I had never used them myself, and that I had no idea what kind of reaction she might have.

This lady was insistent. She looked right at me and demanded, "I am on vacation. I have not enjoyed one single day of this vacation because my sinuses are so clogged up. Let me have some of those berries."

I refused. "You might be allergic."

She couldn't be persuaded. "You said that that man used five. Give me five."

"How about four?" I replied and gave them to her. Then I went to lunch and prayed.

We came back for the afternoon session, and there was that woman sitting in the front row. "You have saved my vacation," she told me.

Since then I have used snowberries to clear the sinuses of two or three other people, with good results. I still would never give them to children or pregnant women because they can be poisonous in quantity, but for healthy adults, four or five berries can work wonders.

White Willow: Billige
Salix species

Old Deer Nose, one of the Crow elders when I was growing up, used to scrape off the top layer of a willow branch and then make a ball of the next wet layer and give it to a person to chew as a headache remedy. He was always giving it to my friends. I guess being my friend gave them a headache.

Willowprine, the aspirin-like substance from willow, is good for a whole list of ailments as a painkiller. I have recommended it to women to take just as soon as they feel a migraine starting. It seems to help.

Editor's Note: The active compound in aspirin, salicylic acid, is named after the Latin name for willow, Salix. Many Native American tribes had been using willow bark as a painkiller for centuries before aspirin was first isolated from it.

Wild Turnip: Ehe
Pediomelum esculentum
Prairie Turnip, Breadroot, Scurf Pea, Timpsula

The best cure for diarrhea and similar intestinal problems, such as irritable bowel syndrome, seems to be a combination of things.

My grandmother always told us not to eat too many wild turnips because they would plug you up. But turnip pablum, in small amounts, was commonly fed to babies. I remembered these two things and thought that turnips must be an effective treatment for diarrhea. It turns out that I was right.

A good friend here in Fort Smith recently had chronic diarrhea. None of the modern medicines would work for more than a day or two. Finally the doctors diagnosed my friend's problem as irritable bowel syndrome, but they had nothing else to give her. I told her to eat turnip flour gruel (just some ground-up dried turnips boiled with a little water), and take it with chokecherry bark and blackberry teas, alternately. (Chokecherry bark taken from the bottom of the tree is the strongest and most effective.)

After two days she started getting better. She has since gained weight and is doing real well. Still, she keeps a jar of turnip flour on hand, just in case.

Spice Rack Remedies

These remedies are not from plants that grow in Montana, but we did have some of them on the spice rack growing up. You probably have a few in your house and might want to grab them when wild plants are not available.

Turmeric helps ease stomachaches and pains. Ginger is great for upset stomachs, dizziness, motion sickness, and the stomach problems that accompany black widow spider bites. Mixing about half a teaspoon of ground ginger in a cup of hot water will make a soothing drink that warms people with colds and settles queasy tummies. Up north they say that a dab of vanilla extract at each temple and along the hair line will keep the gnats away.

My husband drinks fenugreek tea most evenings. It gives him energy and balances his blood sugar. Of course, it's not a traditional plant in this part of the world, but since fenugreek is from India, we can call it an "Old Indian Cure."

7

Other Ways of Healing

Plants do not heal everything. Sometimes we look to the earth or animals for healing cures. Sometimes the power of touch and prayer work. Many of these cures are not rational. I do not know a reason why they work. Still, they have worked, thanks to God, and I do not need to know a reason. I think that sometimes people think too much. They try to find a reason for everything. I try not to question all the time why everything works. I accept that I have a gift for healing, as Pretty Shield did, and I try to use my gift for the best, just as Pretty Shield, who was always giving, did.

Oil for Whooping Cough

When I was seven or eight, old enough to remember, I had whooping cough. The doctors at the clinic couldn't do much for me. They just gave me some cough syrup and maybe some aspirin or some other pill, but that's all. The medicine might have made me stop coughing for a day or two, but it would always come back—a real horrible deep cough.

My grandmother decided that nothing from the clinic was helping. She said, "I will give you something."

She lit a candle and went up among the rafters. We had a bare ceiling, and there in the rafters Pretty Shield hid anything she didn't want us to touch.

She came down with a bottle. It looked to me like an old ketchup bottle with something else in it. She poured a bit into a teaspoon and held it over a candle flame. Of course we didn't have electricity in those days. Nobody did. We used candles in candle stands for light and for heating little bits of things. After the dollop that she had poured into the spoon melted, she cooled it just a little and tested it. Then she brought it over to me and said, "Now put this in your mouth and let it go all over your throat and then swallow it."

So I did.

I still didn't know what it was, but I swallowed it anyway. I always did what she wanted me to. Besides, I didn't like this cough, and Grandma was going to take it away. After that, I quit coughing. It went away.

My sister Mamie was glad that I stopped coughing because she was thinking that I was going to run out of breath. "What did you take?" she asked.

I said, "Grandma gave me something, from up there."

She looked up into the rafters and said, "*Saba?*" That means, "What is it?"

Grandma said, "Skunk oil." (She said it in Crow, of course.)

It was skunk oil. It didn't taste really skunky, yet when I swallowed it, I tasted something that was smart. I didn't care too much for it, but I remember thinking that it wasn't that bad either.

But when Grandma said "skunk oil," I thought, "Boy, I'm cured forever. I don't wanna take that again."

But that's what Pretty Shield did. That's what did it. She knew what she was doing. I have never given anyone skunk oil. I'm not even sure what part of the skunk it was from. But it was very good for curing my whooping cough.

Earth

Special white clay, called *aw wa*, has been used to stop diarrhea. Near where I live, it is found only at the very head of a dry creek bed. The fine powdery clay, a tablespoon or two taken with a little water, really works to check diarrhea. Clay is the stuff that's in Kaopectate, but the Indians were using the special ingredient long before it came in bottles. Also, the white earth mixed with grease and applied to spider bites eases the pain and stops the swelling.

Laying On of Hands

Traditionally there were many kinds of healers in Crow society. Lodgekeepers (homemakers, in other words)—mothers and grandmothers and aunts and wives—did most of the everyday healing. They dealt with cuts and bruises, aches and pains, colds and tummy aches, coughs and bites. The *bajabax ba*, medicine men, dealt with severe physical problems, and some of them worked on spiritual problems as well. Midwives, *ba ain dia auk ha wa sa*, like Pretty Shield, helped deliver babies. And then there were *auk ba pagila*, the pushers.

Once when I was sixteen years old I was working as a nurse's aide in a hospital. A baby with spinal meningitis was brought in from the Cheyenne Reservation. His spine was swayed backward, and his pretty eyes were rolled back. The doctors did everything they could for that baby. Still, that baby just wouldn't eat and wouldn't take any medicines. Nothing. He was just bent backward.

I was assigned to that room, to clean up and keep the baby's sheets clean. The baby was wrapped up in a bunting; he was that small. I felt so sorry for this little bitty baby. Finally I asked the doctor if I couldn't ask a pusher to come. She was a praying woman, a Christian one, really, but she still had her ways, her old ways.

He said, "There is nothing we can do for him, Alma. Go ahead."

The mother had already left. She couldn't stand to see her baby die. Her sister was to stay with that little baby until it died. I asked the aunt, and she said, "Go ahead."

And so I went to Libby Bear Cloud, who was a healer. I told her that I would buy her groceries—meat and stuff like that—because she was really poor. Most of us were poor, but the older ones, like Libby, they had nothing, and they couldn't do anything to make money.

So Libby said she would push the baby. She came to the hospital and told me, "Stand at the door. Don't let anybody in. And I want the aunt out of here too."

I stood outside the door but left it cracked a little bit. Libby washed her hands in the restroom. She came out, and I saw that she had olive oil with her. She took the baby and unwrapped it. The baby was still swayed back. Libby took the baby on her lap, put a sheet on herself, and poured the oil on the baby.

She poured the oil all over his body, even on the bottom of his feet, everywhere. Then she started to massage the baby. Libby started talking in a language I didn't know. I was a Baptist girl, and they never ever spoke in what they call tongues in that church. I peeked in the hospital room, and there she was talking in this language and rubbing him and rubbing him and rubbing him. Finally she stopped and wrapped up the baby. She wrapped him the way we wrap Indian babies. She put him in the little crib, and she went and washed up. I opened the door, and she said, "The baby will live. But I have to come four times. I have three more times left. Come pick me up, and I'll come."

After that first time with Libby the baby began to limber up a little bit. After the second time he was even better. After the third time he was eating rice water. The fourth time she came, Libby said, "The baby is well." And so he was.

The doctor, he said, "Amazing." He said, "It's a miracle." He said, "Thank you, Alma," because he too was glad the baby lived.

And so this little baby was taken home, and I was happy.

One day I went to my grandma's little house in Crow Agency, and this group of people came up. They were carrying gifts; it was this little baby's parents.

I said, "I don't want any gifts. Please don't give me anything. If you have to give them to somebody, give them to Libby. She needs these things."

"Well," they said, "we want you to have something too. We know it was you who went after Libby." They put a bracelet on me, a silver one. It was so pretty. A minute later, off my wrist it came. One of my nieces who was just becoming a teenager jerked it off and took it, but that didn't make me flinch a bit.

The parents took the other gifts over to Libby. She was very happy.

"You have blessed me," she said. "You blessed me."

The parents replied, "They're not equivalent to the blessing that you have brought us because our baby is alive."

I recently told my sister this story. She reminded me about a neighbor of hers. "There's a middle-aged man, now, living way up there around Lame Deer, Montana. He limps just a little bit."

I believe that's him. That's that little baby, all grown up.

Personal Pushing Experience

I am not an *auk ba pagila*, a pusher, like Libby Bear Cloud was, but I have helped people heal through touch and prayer.

A few years back a young man came to the house. He was working for the National Park Service down at Yellowtail Dam, which is only two miles away. This man was hurting in his kidneys and back.

A bunch of people were sitting around the house, but I told him to drop his pants anyway. He leaned against the fridge and then he lowered his pants down and pushed his shirt up. I laid my hands on him, on both sides of where he was hurting, in the kidney area and the back. I began that pushing, and I said a prayer.

A few minutes later the pain was easing. "Mmmmmm," he said, "Thank you. Is that all? What do I owe you?"

I answered, "Nothing. Just get well."

Then he went. "Thank you."

You know, he said his back hasn't bothered him since.

I don't know how. But it happens.

Another time a pregnant woman who lived in Fort Smith came to the house while I was talking to two young people in the living room. The woman was sweating and crying. "My baby's going to be breach," she told us. "I came here to ask for your prayers."

I told her I would pray for her, and I asked her to sit down.

I talked to the baby while the other two people prayed, and the woman, she just sat there afraid with her unmoving baby.

I put my hands or her stomach and felt around. Then I told that baby, "Quit being lazy! Just turn."

Suddenly there was this big ball of something sticking up on the woman's side. A fist or something. Then there was a big movement inside, and the woman felt better.

We said some more prayers and sent her to the doctor right away. After all that movement inside, she wanted to know what had happened.

The doctor asked her, "What did you do? The baby is much better. It's in the right position."

She replied, "I went to see Alma Snell, and Alma Snell went to her Lord Jesus."

Thoughts on Healing

Young pushers are rare these days. Almost no Crow children grow up to be midwives or healers. I think this is because healing involves more than giving somebody a back rub or picking a few herbs. It needs to be very solemn. Healing is a building up of faith and meditation. Then you must always be in the right mood because you know that at any time anyone might call on you. You don't want to be doing something that is out of the path when you must help someone. That's the reason so many young people don't learn these things. Their minds might think, "Oh my, that's beautiful; I want to do that," but they are out of their realm. To get into the right realm takes time and effort. To be a healer you need to be in the Kingdom Realm.

Obedience and Patience

Healing requires more than a good healer and the right herbs. Of course, faith is important, but so is the right attitude from the patient.

People are always calling me and saying, "Alma, my doctor told me to do this or that, and it's too hard. What can you give me instead?" They seem surprised when I tell them to follow their doctor's instructions. Most of the time doctors know what they are doing, and besides, there is power in obedience.

When your doctor or nurse advises you about what to do and what not to do, stick to it. Be obedient. Obedience is power. It will make you healthy. It will make you happy. Maybe it will make you better. Listen. Be obedient.

Patience is also powerful. Sometime you don't want to wait. Sometimes it just seems too long and too hard. But with the Lord's help, you can wait. Don't take the short route about anything. If you can be patient and obedient, you'll be better for it. Then you'll win the battle.

When the Body Doesn't Heal

Sometimes the body is past repair. That should not be a problem as long as you are right with the Creator.

Recently a woman called, tired and weeping, "Alma, my husband is dying, and it just seems that we're sitting here waiting."

I said to her, "Be happy for him. I see the gates opening up. It's opening up for the redeemed, and there is joy in walking toward those gates. He doesn't want you to be too sorrowful. Be happy that he is walking in the light."

His ways are not ours, and our ways are not His. Still, I know that the creator of all time did not make us so just to end. There is much jubilation as people leave this life and walk through those gates of light. We cannot know what awaits us. I know it is more.

I hope that these remedies help you to have a happy and healthy life here on earth. I also hope that you know love and joy and pass it on, for this life and the next.

Follow Your Own Path

I remind people that whatever they're gifted in, they should stay in that realm.

It's that way, I think. It's that way with everything. I think that you can be skilled at everything and a master of nothing. Don't do that. If you're needed in a certain category, stay in that category and make the most of it and help people. That's what we're here for, to help one another. If we don't help each other, what's the use of living?

Living just to enjoy myself, have a good time, and then die without doing something for my fellow man is a complete waste of time.

That's what I believe. It might be my own philosophy, and I may be wrong, but I do think that it has helped me help people.

PART THREE

Beauty and Love

Eating well and being healthy are the most important ways to look good. Still, it seems that at the Taste of Heritage programs I give, people always perk up when I start talking about beauty and love. Everyone seems to be looking to put a little extra spark in their life, a glow on their cheeks, or a sparkle in their eyes. Here are a few of my secrets.

8

Beauty Secrets

Every morning when she was cooking breakfast outside her lodge, my Grandmother Pretty Shield would look out at the other women around the camp and notice how nice they looked. She'd look at one, and if her hair was really nicely braided, all smooth and neat, then she knew that woman was well taken care of by her husband. Here and there she'd see one with bushy hair or one whose braids had little pieces of hair sticking out. Those women's husbands didn't look after them so well. Looking good represented more than just vanity.

While baking bread or some other food, she would look over the camp and categorize everyone to herself. She would think, "That one isn't loved very much," and "That one really is loved."

I asked her, "Did Grandpa do your hair real good?"

"Always," she said. "Always," and she smiled.

I don't have long braids, and my hair is not always the neatest, but I have learned some tricks over the years to help people look their best. Here I have included some instructions for using the earth's cosmetics, some historical beauty tips, and some modern tricks for using plants to look your best.

Everyday Hygiene

Cold Water Secrets

Bathing in cold water was important to the Crow people. Cold water is stimulating and makes people shiver, which makes them sweat. It also makes a person tough.

When we lived in Black Lodge, Bill would drive to work along the Little Big Horn River early each morning. Every day, even in the middle of winter, there'd be this old man sitting in the river. In winter, he would be sitting in a hole that he'd cut in the ice. He wore a big ten-gallon hat, and he'd wave at Bill as he passed.

I don't know of anyone who does that any more. In the winter I go outside and sit in my hot tub and come out steaming. But then, back in the time of Plenty Coups, warriors needed to be able to ride on horseback from Fort Livingstone (in Saskatchewan)to Fort Belknap just to spy on the other tribes. They had no choice but to be tough. I can ride in a car.

Skin Care

Among Indian women, I think wrinkles come mostly from facing the harsh weather. Old women with shriveled faces will have soft, smooth arms because they always wore long sleeves and their arms were protected from the sun and wind. Staying out of sweat lodges also helps prevent wrinkles.

To prevent sunburn, old ladies would mix red earth with grease and rub it on themselves. Bill's grandma, One Woman, used to do that all the time, even if she was wearing a brand new dress. She'd mix red earth with tallow and rub it all over her neck. She would deliberately dust red earth all over the dress from the waist up. Every neckline of every dress that she had turned a dusty red after just one wearing.

Collecting the right red earth takes some doing. Not just any red sand will do. You must dig it from way deep, where the sun and the oxygen can't reach it. Back in there the earth has a different smell and consistency from regular soil. To get it, you need to find a deep crevice, and then get a long strong stick—usually a willow or chokecherry branch—and stick it in as far as you can. Bring it out. If you use the red earth soon, it doesn't need to be mixed with tallow, but it does last longer when it's mixed. Besides making a great sunscreen, this type of earth also makes a fine rouge and can be mixed with buffalo grease to make a long-lasting war paint.

To care for our lips in the sun and the wind, we would look for cooling plants. Mint tea, made from *Mentha arvensis*, was the best, and it grew right along the river's edge where we were anyway. We'd mix the mint with tallow to keep our lips greasy. The mixture cooled them and kept them from drying out and cracking.

Crow clans are named after some characteristic trait. Grandma's clan was Greasy Mouth. Some say that the name came from having plenty of good things to eat. I think it's more likely that the clan was called Greasy Mouth from our being out in the sun so much and putting the minty tallow on our lips.

Crow women traditionally never wore hats. Assiniboine women did, but Crow women covered their heads with scarves. These days, with all we know about skin cancer, I recommend that everyone who works outside wear sunscreen and a hat that shades the face. If you do get sunburned, rubbing on yarrow tea will help ease the burning and prevent blistering and peeling.

Teeth

Cooled cinders were used to clean the teeth. My sister Cerise scrubbed her mouth with charcoal, and she had nice teeth. At my house, before toothbrushes were common, we'd just rinse out our mouths really well and gargle, first thing in the morning.

Later the clinics gave us toothbrushes and told us to use them with baking soda. We did that most of the time. We liked toothpaste too, when we could get it, but it wasn't always available and could be expensive. Most of the time we just used soda.

A single section of horsetail (*Equisetum* species) makes a good tooth scrubber. The plant contains a lot of silica, which helps grind off stuck-on food. We also sometimes used thorns from hawthorn trees (*Crataegus* species) as toothpicks.

Cosmetics

Nature provides bountiful cosmetics. Traditionally Crow women seldom made cosmetics. Women cleaned their faces, greased them with

BEAUTY AND LOVE

buffalo grease for moisture, and sometimes wore blush, but it was the men who really painted their faces. They mixed their own colors and painted their faces for war and special ceremonies.

Red and orange colors were made from red earth that has not been exposed to the sun. Red earth seems to be a face lifter. It makes people look younger and healthier. Charcoal was used for darkening eyebrows. Other colors were made from plants. Elderberries and juneberries were used for blues and purples. Juneberries really stain. They make the best, longest-lasting paint. Grass was used for greens, while goldenrod flowers made a nice golden yellow.

To make paint, collect the berries, grass, or flowers for the color you want. Boil the plant material with a little water and some buffalo hooves. The gelatinous substance from the hooves makes the paint thick and shiny. Spread the colored mixture over a rawhide to dry. When it is dried, break it up into little pieces with a stick. Place the pieces in a little sack, putting a little of the color on the top flap so you know what color it contains without needing to open it.

When you are ready to use the paint, open the sack, take out some pieces, and heat them a little to melt them into a spreadable paste. You're ready to paint. Gloss over your work with a little more gel from buffalo hooves if you are going for a really moist look.

I learned from Bill's people, the Assiniboine, that porcupine quills are dyed using these same plants. Porcupine quills are used to decorate many things. The quills are soaked in the plant mixture, but I never learned this old way. Modern women use Rit brand dye.

Speaking of porcupine quills and beauty, Lena Blue Robe Snell pierced my ears with porcupine quills. She soaked the quills in an alcohol solution, washed my ears with alcohol, started the quills in my ear lobes, and then she cut the quills in half. She had also tied my hair back. On the third day, she pulled the quill through carefully with a tweezers. Then she inserted a sanitized gold wire, and it worked very well.

Skin Problems

Dry Skin and Rashes

Aubon ba a ba la, evening primrose oil (from *Oenothera biennis*), works well for skin problems like dryness, eczema, and rashes. It also works as a soothing everyday moisturizer, and taking it internally helps nourish skin from the inside.

Crow women traditionally extract the oil from the flowers using water. Pick a bunch of evening primrose flowers, just cover them with water, and simmer gently for twenty minutes. Let the mixture sit until all the water evaporates. Strain off the flowers and use the oil that's left behind. Now, you can also buy evening primrose oil in health-food stores. If you can't find it in liquid form, you can probably buy it in gel capsules. Poke the end of the capsule with a needle and spread the oil on the infected skin.

Chemotherapy can cause hideous-looking rashes and breakouts on the face and other parts of the body. I recommended that a friend rub evening primrose oil along with vitamin E oil directly on her rashes. It didn't take long for her skin to clear up. Old Indian remedies can be applied to new problems.

Dirty or Oily Skin

Indian women long ago used mud for soap. They'd cake it on, and when they rinsed it off, all the dirt and impurities went with it. They were way ahead of their time, what with these mud masks that you can get at a spa now.

Skunkbush tonic is a great astringent for tightening the pores and leaving your face glowing. The *ba yew hish she sih shea*, skunkbush (*Rhus aromatica*, a plant I sometimes call bitterbush) is a small shrub that grows on the slopes of the foothills. The berries are ruddy orange and somewhat hairy. The leaves smell slightly skunky, and the berries taste acidic and fresh.

I keep a little jar of skunkbush tonic with me when I give programs on traditional plant uses. I ask for a volunteer, and I wash her face with the skunkbush berry tonic. I make sure that the whole audience sees

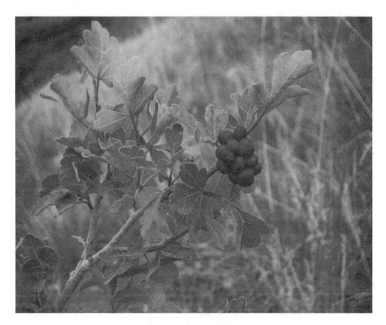

Skunkbush

her before and after. The change is amazing. It tightens up the face and makes it look glossy and healthy.

☙ Skunkbush Tonic

> Collect ripe or slightly dried berries of the skunkbush (*Rhus aromatica*). Cover them with water and simmer for 20 minutes. Then mash the mixture, squeezing all the juice out of the berries. Let the mixture settle. Decant and use the liquid.

Besides serving well an astringent, this skunkbush tonic also helps ease the pain of bites and poison ivy rashes. A little boy who lives near here got into some poison ivy, and a rash broke out on his face. It was so bad that he could hardly sleep, but it was nighttime, and his family didn't want to drive all the way to Crow Agency, where the hospital is. I gave them some skunkbush tonic and told them to soak cheesecloth in it and hold it to his face. They did that, and that little boy slept all night. The next day his family took him to the doctor in Crow, but he was already well on his way to healing.

Warts

After the first thunder in the spring, pick some green grass, spit on it, and rub it on your warts until they turn green. They'll go away right after that, or so Pretty Shield always told me, and I've seen it work.

Herbalists tell me that the milky sap from milkweed (*Asclepias* species) helps to eliminate warts too. Just break the stem and rub the milk onto the wart.

Editor's Note: After Alma told me Pretty Shield's cure for warts, Alma's husband, Bill, told me, "Prevention is the best cure for warts."

Intrigued, I asked, "How do you prevent warts?"

"Stay away from toads," he replied.

Hair Care

Old-Fashioned Hair Care Tips

Rainwater is the best water for washing and rinsing hair.

Sage (*Artemesia* species) and iron, boiled together, is good for darkening hair and eyebrows, and you don't need to worry about your gray roots showing. I've never used it myself, but I'm sure this solution is a lot better for you than these chemicals they use to dye hair these days.

Porcupine-quill brushes were thought to be the best hairbrushes. They work better than bone or stick combs and leave the hair shiny.

Indian women always braided their hair, not only to keep it neat and out of their faces but also because they say that braiding it every night before bed makes it grow faster.

Scrubbing sand into long hair leaves it fantastically shiny. It sounds strange, but it really works. When I was growing up, most of the time we would bathe in a nearby stream. We'd use whatever soap we had for washing everything, including our hair, and then we'd rinse in the river. The older girls, those with long beautiful hair, would scrub their hair with sand and then rinse it out real well. They'd feel it and if there were any sand left, they'd get back in the water and let the stream carry it away. When it dried, it was really shiny. In the old days men also used sand rinses. Then after their hair was clean, they'd spread it out on a large sunny rock and sit and chat while their hair dried.

Beaver oil gives hair great shine too. In the old days, the Crows would rub beaver oil on the scalp and then wrap the head for a while, sometimes even for days. The water and oils trapped under the wrapping would really moisturize the hair. It would come out thick, strong, and really shiny. I never tried wrapping my head like that, but I think Pretty Shield probably brushed some of that oil into our hair when we were little.

Sweetgrass (*bachuate*, *Hierchloe odorata*) makes a great after-shampoo rinse. Boil some sweetgrass in water and let it cool. After shampooing your hair, rinse it with the sweetgrass tea. Your hair will become thick and healthy.

When I was growing up, one boy at my school had beautiful, thick shiny black hair. We knew his family was poor, so they couldn't have been spending any money on fancy hair products. Finally he revealed his secret: Crisco mixed with Blue Waltz perfume.

Eating the entrails and innards of animals, especially the stomach, which are the parts highest in protein, will help your hair grow thick and strong.

Rinsing with a tea of greasewood (*Baashesshehpiia*, *Cercocarpus ledifolius*, also known as mountain mahogany) can be used against lice.

Baldness Cure

I know a nurse who started getting a little bald spot near the top of her head, and nothing seemed to help make the hair grow back. She went to a Crow man. He told her to use yucca root (*oox' ish baut shua*, *Yucca glauca*) and to split the root with the grain instead of across it. She was to apply a sudsy yucca tea made from the split root to the bald spot and just keep applying it. She did, and the hair grew back. She had her full head of hair again.

Awhile later when a man in town came to me because he was starting to lose his hair, I knew just what to try. I gave him the yucca and told him to put it on his head and leave it there for a little while. By the third day he was all excited. There was a little bit of fuzz growing on the edges of the bald spot.

But then his wife, with a really repulsed face, asked, "Steve, what is that I smell on you?"

He explained, and proudly showed her the little fuzz.

She only scowled, "Sure smells. I can't stand that smell."

"Well, would you rather that I smell for a while and end up with a full head of hair or have this bald spot?" he asked.

She didn't wait to answer. "I'll take you bald."

Fragrance

Creating Good Smells

Crow women I have known, when they were working hard on crafts or other projects, would put some flowers—something good smelling like roses or dame's rocket—in a little bowl on the table. Every once in a while, while they were working, they'd just reach over and run their hands through the petals to get the smell, and they would feel better. They call this aromatherapy now, and people think it is a new "alternative" therapy, but really people have been enjoying fragrance for centuries. Back then it gave them a sense of feeling better, just as it does now.

Pretty Shield put sweet pine on the hot flat surface of her woodburning stove, and the smoke would fill the house. She'd do it just for the smell. It was cleansing to have that fragrance all over you. Sometimes I'll go around the house just making cleansing smoke. Bill has to hide in the back room while I go through with burning pine, sage, and sweetgrass.

Covering Bad Smells

Foot Odor

Soaking your feet for a while in buffalo blood is supposed to remedy stinky feet. I have no personal experience of doing this, but if you want to try it, I'm sure that it will work.

Besides soaking your feet in blood, if you want to get rid of foot odor you can try using cool mint tea. Soak your feet in the tea for quite a while. Keep soaking them twice a week for three weeks and see what happens. It can't hurt.

Or you could try sage and cedar. Flat sage (*Artemisia ludoviciana*) is also supposed to do wonders for bad smells. Mix the sage with sweet cedar (*Juniperus scopulorum*), brew it, mix it with clay to make mud, and pack your feet in the mud. Just sit there and relax for the afternoon. When you remove the mud, it should take the dirt and the odors with it. Sage and pine both draw out smells and toxins and leave their own nice fragrance.

Body Odor

The purple flowers of the Canadian thistles (*Cirsium* species) supposedly work against stinky body odors. One gentleman, Phillip White Clay (he's a little older than I am), said that he treated a woman with tea made from thistle flowers. She just splashed the tea under her arms—washed and splashed it on, washed and splashed it on. Finally she got rid of the bad part of her sweating, her bad body odor.

Tea made from Canadian thistles checked it. I have never tried this myself. I have no idea what thistle smells like in tea, but I believe it works.

Meanwhile, a little fresh mint will do a lot for bad breath. Even a glass of mint tea helps. So does chewing on fresh rose petals.

Attitude: The Secret to Staying Young

My grandson Erik is a pharmacist over at the clinic at Crow Agency. Every time I go over there for a checkup, I guess all the ladies who live in Crow ask Erik how old I am. When he tells them that I'm eighty-two, they ask for my secrets for how I look so young. He tells them that I rub lemon juice on my face, which I sometimes do. The truth is, though, I don't think I look that young. But I do feel good, and I guess I look good for an old lady.

Only I don't think I'm an old lady. That's the real secret. You look and feel as old as you act, and I don't have time to act like an old lady. I laugh a lot, I eat well, I pray, and I always have something to do. That keeps me young.

9

Love Medicines

Crow people have long been known as passionate lovers, and every once in a while I'm told that I am a "Love Mama" among these passionate people. I don't know quite what that means, but I have never seemed to have trouble getting attention from males. (Sometimes I have received far too much attention, but you can read about that in my book *Grandmother's Grandchild*.) Of course, when you live a long life, you have a chance to see most everything, and I have a lifetime of advice to give. From flirting to attraction to pregnancy, here's what this Crow Love Mama has to say.

Flirting

When we were growing up, young ladies weren't allowed to attract attention in many ways, but chewing gum was one method we could use. We'd chew gum from the clear sap of young pine trees. It used to be quite the thing to smack it just right. If you could do it rhythmically—pop it every other bite—that was really good. It was considered kind of sexy but acceptable. Popping was a way to get people to notice you. It said, "I'm sexy and available." The men sang a good song about the women chewing gum, but they had another song they sang if a girl was acting too silly in front of the guys: "You've got dandy hightop moccasins; why don't you go elsewhere?"

While popping gum was quite the thing on the reservation, if we were at school or anywhere off the reservation, the matrons would tell us it was rude. We'd have to stop and act more "ladylike," but once we were back on the reservation, we could pop gum while acting like a lady.

Aphrodisiacs

Different aphrodisiac items were special to different Crow families, and some things used by one weren't even thought of by another family. Beaver musk was the scent of allure to Pretty Shield. She created a family necklace that consists of sky blue beads with four red beads on four strands, two on each side. Next to the red beads are elk teeth (for the girls only), and in the middle are dried beaver castors, the source of the musk (for the boys). She fixed those necklaces (without the musk) for her daughters and granddaughters when they were young women, before they were married. That was the family necklace we had to attract good husbands. I didn't get one, however. By the time I came around, it was hard to find real elk teeth and especially hard to get beaver castors. Still, beaver musk is supposed to be the scent of allure, for men anyway. The sacredness of any necklace in a family was well respected.

When I met Bill, I had no thought of charms. That type of stuff suddenly vanished. The Assiniboine love medicine must have overpowered all other ways. (Grandmother was right on to this Assiniboine spell mentioned in *Grandmother's Grandchild*.)

For those who do not have access to beaver musk, I recommend *egish gigeshepita hisha*, elkweed, for serious love seekers. Just rub some of the dried leaves on your hands, rub a bit on the person you want to attract, and walk away. Someone will follow you, I guarantee it. Sometimes a honeymoon follows too.

Elkweed (*Ceanothus velutinus*), sometimes called red root, is a short bush that grows in wet places in the mountains west of here. A sprig of its dried leaves can work wonders. It is strong, potent. We should call it "obsession." People become obsessed with you when you wear it. I tease people about it, but it really can be used like a fancy perfume.

At one presentation in Billings, I was talking about elkweed when a cowboy insisted that I give him some. I said, "Sure, take some." I had a big box of it at the time. I didn't know how well it would really work, but it is a nice sensation for the senses.

The next year I was presenting again at the college in Billings. A man raised his hand while I was talking about elkweed, and I thought, "That one looks kind of familiar."

As soon as he stood up and started to speak, I recognized him as the cowboy who took all the elkweed. He came up to the front and announced, "This really works. I used the elkweed last year and since then I married the one I wanted."

I smiled, "Oh, dear."

He told the crowd how well it worked. Boy, everyone in the audience gathered around to try it.

Elkweed also charms married couples. My friend Robyn is an herbalist over in Bozeman. Every year for many years she would leave her husband, Tom, in Montana and take off for herb classes in Arizona. Poor Tom was always here working while she was down there learning more about plants for weeks and weeks at a time, every year.

I was feeling sorry for Tom, always here, working away, all alone. So I gave him a little sprig of elkweed and told him to put it under her pillow.

The next year Bill and I were eating dinner with Robyn and Tom. She was telling me about all the things she had learned in Arizona, and I asked, "Well, Robyn, are you going to go down there again this year?"

She looked around, picked at her food, and said, "Well, I don't think so. I feel so sorry for Tom. He works so hard. He needs me, Alma. I think I'd better not leave him again."

I looked over at Tom. When Robyn looked down to take the next bite of her dinner, he smiled and pulled a sprig of elkweed out of his pocket. It works.

We have fun with that elkweed. You can smell it all over at some powwows. Elk love it too, in case you were wondering. They nibble on the blossoms, and it just drives them crazy. Yes, they nibble on those elkweed flowers and all of a sudden they have this uncontrollable urge. They can't stop themselves. A few bites of that elkweed and those big bull elk just have to stand up and whistle.

If you want to engage in more than just innocent flirting, take some clear pine sap used for chewing gum and mix it with prairie onions (*Allium* species). Then you watch out, boy. You'd just better behave yourself too. The wild onions are more like garlic than onions. Like garlic, the smell stays with you, and it sure is a strange-tasting combination. But if you ever want to get a jolting start to your young life, you just keep eating that, a little onion mixed with that clear sap as a gum. It's a strong aphrodisiac, and some say it helps with impotence too.

To Get Pregnant

In many books you can read that stone seed (*Lithospermum ruderale*) works as a contraceptive. I know of a woman who used it, but it worked too well. She could never have children after using it. The Crow word for stone seed, *eldocxabio*, means "miscarriage plant." I don't mess with it. It's too touchy. The wrong dose can leave a woman sterile. Besides, the women who come to me all want help getting pregnant. They want babies, not the other way around.

If wild onions haven't worked to help a woman get pregnant, I usually tell her to eat foods like soy, which mimics estrogen, and to also go to the Lord with prayers. One time I told a woman of another technique that I had learned from a tribe in Washington State. She was to make a small fire and throw a little sweet pine and sage incense on the coals. Then she was to spread her legs and stand over the fire, using her garments as a tent to let that incense smoke swirl around her legs. She was of another tribe, so I never heard back from her, but I think it worked. Perhaps if you try, believing, it will work.

Secrets for a Long Marriage

"What do you recommend for broken hearts?" asked Lisa, my editor.

"Elkweed," I answered. "If your 'love' still leaves you, the person was never yours anyway. Go and find someone who is truly yours." I don't have much to say about that kind of broken heart.

Sometimes, though, I see broken hearts in marriages. Most of these can be avoided. Bill and I have been married for more than fifty years through some really hard times. I have learned a few things during that time.

You get married because you really love the person, and vice versa. You have so much fun being lovers. It's wonderful. Then, usually after the kids come along, it's harder. At those times people need to remember that when they get married, they really marry three people: 1) a lover, 2) a friend, and 3) a brother or sister.

In order to be the best wife or husband you can be, you need to be: 1) a lover, 2) a friend, and 3) a brother or sister. The trick is to apply all three at the right time. Doing that really seems to patch a family together.

I tell women that sometimes your husband will need you to be a friend. He will need you to give advice, tell him when he's right and when he's wrong, and listen to what he has to say, as a friendly companion. During some of the harder times, your husband will need you to be a sister. He will need you to comfort and forgive and pray with him. At these times, you can be in the family of the Great Spirit and allow His grace to help you, and you can leave your problems in His hands.

Soon the time will come again when you are lovers. You are happy just to be in each other's arms and you are husband and wife. You can go away together and leave this world for a while and be part of a spiritual world. You knit your family together spiritually.

It takes all three to make a marriage last: lovers, friends, and brothers and sisters. The trick is knowing when to be each. I hope you can figure it out for your relationships.

Conclusion

Food, medicine, beauty, and love. When we talk about them in English, they seem so different from each other. But looking at them from another perspective, they are not so different. Good food is a part of good health. Good health leads to good looks. Love surrounds it all. When we feed or heal, we share love. When we love and are loved, we are beautiful.

God has provided for us food and medicine. We are loved. God's creation is a beautiful system. We just need to learn to take a look around and listen carefully because there is still so much to learn about the wonders that surround us. This book is a start. I pray that you will continue to learn and walk with the magnificence of nature. When nature heals you, you have discovered nature.

When I started giving presentations, my sister Pearl Hogan reminded me, "Just be sure you are genuine about what you do. It is a good adventure to dig, not only *ehe*, the wild turnip roots, but also the knowledge of grandmother and the other elders who taught us to survive on God's provisions. All it takes is work. It's up to you. My prayers are always with you."

It is still an adventure to dig into the knowledge of those who have gone before. It is work. But, readers, it is up to you. My prayers are with you.

Appendix

PLANT LIST

English Name	Crow Name	Scientific Name	Alternative Name(s)
Arrowleaf balsamroot	Augaurashkose seega	Balsamorrhiza sagittata	
Bear root	Esa	Lomatium disticum	
Bitterroot	Basauxawa	Lewisia rediviva	
Box elder	Bishpe	Acer negundo	
Buffaloberry	Baishhesha	Sheperdia canadensis	Bullberry
Burdock root		Arctium minus	
Camas root	Basashbita upbooba lusua	Cammassia quamash	
Cattails	Baxosa	Typha species	
Cedar berry	Baga eli gee chia bagua	Juniperus horizontalis	Creeping juniper
Chokecherry	Baju dala	Prunus virginiana	
Corn (silk)	Xoxashegia	Zea mays	
Dandelion	Ba oohba she lay	Taraxacum officinalis	
Echinacea	Egigeshishibita	Echinacea angustifolia	Black root, snake root, purple coneflower
Elderberry	Balawoolatebagua	Sambucus racemosa	Hollowwood berry
Elkweed	Egish gigeshepita hisha	Ceanothus velutinus	Red root
Evening primrose	Aubon ba a ba la	Oenothera biennis	
Flax	Esshogebalia	Linum species; Linum lewisii (blue flax)	
Gooseberries and currants	Be ga ge ta	Ribes species	
Grapes	Dax bee chay ish ta shay	Vitus species	Slick bears' eyes
Greasewood	Baashesshehpiia	Cercocarpus ledifolius	Mountain mahogany

English Name	Crow Name	Scientific Name	Alternative Name(s)
Ground tomato	Bitgup awada	Physalis pumila	Wild tomatillo, husk tomato, ground cherry
Hawthorns	Beelee chi sha yeah	Crataegus species	
Horsetail	Auxbawlax ecoosua	Equisetum species	Joint weed, ghost pipe
Huckleberries	Kapi:lia:zde	Vaccinium species	
Indian lettuce	Becashua ba luasua	Montia species	Miner's lettuce
Indian paintbrush	Ba abali chi gua gat tay	Castilleja species	
Juneberry	Bacu wu lete	Amelanchier alnifolia	Serviceberry, sarviceberry, saskatoon, shad bush
Kinnikinnick	Obeezia	Arctostaphylos uva-ursi	Bearberry
[Lichen]	A wa ga chilua	Xanthoptimelia chlorchroa	
Little peppergrass	Bicaw eshia	Lepidium species	
Mint	Shushue	Mentha arvensis	
Monarda	Aw wa xom bilish bi baba	Monarda fistulosa	Bee balm, mountain mint
Sphagnum moss	Bee ma ga sut che	Sphagnum species	
Mullein	Aubeesay	Verbascum thapsus	
Nettles	Babaliatocha	Urtica dioica	
Oregon grape	Away daubish bagua	Mahonia repens	Creeping mahonia, grape holly
Pennycress	Chate ishbitaba bagoota	Thlaspi arvense	
Pennyroyal	Chate ishbeleeshbita	Hedeoma hispida	Coyote mint
Pincushion cactus	Bitchgalee bajua	Coryphantha species	
Plantain	Begeelish aubalay	Plantago virginicum	
Ponderosa pine	Bageeah	Pinus ponderosa	
Prairie coneflower	Awa chu geba aba lee sheela	Ratibida columnifera	Mexican hat
Prickly pear cactus	Bitchgalee baaba lee gish sha	Opuntia species	
Purple prairie clover	Awa chu geba a balee shee la	Dalea purpurea	

English Name	Crow Name	Scientific Name	Alternative Name(s)
Raspberries	Baaxuaga	Rubus species	
Roses	Bijaba	Rosa species	
Sage	Esushgexuwa	Artemesia species	
Salsify	Ba boba sheeb dauxa	Tragopogon dubius	Oyster plant, goatsbeard
Saw grass		Spartina pectinata	Prairie cord grass
Sego lilies	Minmo baba leegisha	Calochortus species	
Shepherd's purse	Awa xoshshebit	Capsella bursa-pastoris	
Showy milkweed		Asclepias speciosa	
Skunkbush	Ba yew hish she sih shea	Rhus armomatica	
Snowberry	Bitdaja	Symphoricarpus occidentalis	
Squash	Coogooehsa		
Stoneseed	Eldocxabio	Lithospermum ruderale	Miscarriage plant
Sweetgrass	Bachuate	Hierchloe odorata	
White willow	Billige	Salix species	
Wild asparagus	Sow ba she shesh peah	Asparagus officinalis	
Wild carrot	Bikka:sahte	Perideridia gairdneri	Split root, yampa, squaw root
Wild onions	Bitxua	Allium textile and other Allium species	
Wild Plum	Buluhpe	Prunus americana	
Wild turnip	Ehe	Pediomelum esculentum	Prairie turnips, bread root, scurf pea
Yarrow	Chibaapooshchishgota	Achillea millefolium	Chipmunk tail
Yucca	Oox'ish bautshua	Yucca glauca	Deer's awl

References

I hope this "taste" of some Crow heritage leaves you wanting to know more. This list includes the books that I've mentioned in the chapters, a few of the many great ethnobotanical books I like to read, and my favorite flower identification books.

Duke, James A. *The Green Pharmacy*. Emmaus PA: Rodale Press, 1997.

Kindscher, Kelly. *Edible Wild Plants of the Prairie: An Ethnobotanical Guide*. Lawrence: University Press of Kansas, 1987.

———. *Medicinal Wild Plants of the Prairie: An Ethnobotanical Guide*. Lawrence: University Press of Kansas, 1992.

Krumm, Bob, and James Krumm. *The Pacific Northwest Berry Book*. Helena MT: Falcon Press, 1998.

Le Draoulec, Pascale. *American Pie: Slices of Life (and Pie) from America's Back Roads*. New York: Harper Collins, 2002.

Linderman, Frank B. 1932. *Pretty-Shield: Medicine Woman of the Crows*. Reprinted with a preface by Alma Snell and Becky Matthews. Lincoln: University of Nebraska Press, 2003.

McCleary, Timothy P. "Apsáalooke Plant List." Unpublished, prepared for Little Big Horn College, 2004.

Medicine Horse, Mary Helen. *A Dictionary of Everyday Crow*. Crow Agency MT: Bilingual Materials Development Center, 1987.

Phillips, H. Wayne. *Central Rocky Mountain Wildflowers*. Helena MT: Falcon Press, 1999.

Snell, Alma Hogan. *Grandmother's Grandchild: My Crow Indian Life*. Edited by Becky Matthews. Lincoln: University of Nebraska Press, 2000.

Spellenberg, Richard. *National Audubon Society Field Guide to North American Wildflowers*. New York: Alfred A. Knopf, 1979.

Tilford, Gregory. *Edible and Medicinal Plants of the West*. Missoula: Montana Press Publishing Company, 1997.

Willard, Terry. *Edible and Medicinal Plants of the Rocky Mountain and Neighbouring Territories*. Calgary AB: Wild Rose College of Natural Healing, 1992.

Index

Good Things
Jane Grigson

Dining with Marcel Proust
A Practical Guide to French
Cuisine of the Belle Epoque
Shirley King
Foreword by James Beard

Pampille's Table
Recipes and Writings from the
French Countryside from
Marthe Daudet's
Les Bons Plats de France
Translated and adapted by Shirley King